ABOUT THE AUTHOR

Professor Valery Feigin, MD, MSc, PhD is currently neurologist and Senior Research Fellow at the University of
Auckland. A founding member and past chairman of two
scientific panels of the European Federation of Neurological
Societies, he has written over 150 scientific articles on
various aspects of stroke, including contributions to a WHO
handbook. He has worked at the Mayo Clinic in the United
States, and in the University Department of Neurology at
Utrecht University in the Netherlands.

He has written four textbooks, and one of his books,
Handbook of Stroke, co-written with D.O. Wiebers and R.D.
Brown Jr, has been translated into several languages.

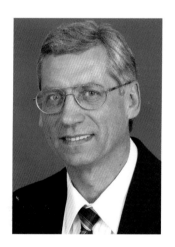

D1546902

More about the book

This is a remarkable book in that it covers almost every aspect of stroke from its prevention through to caring for a stroke patient. I strongly recommend it to all general readers, particularly to the many who have been either directly or indirectly touched by stroke.

Professor Geoffrey Donnan
National Stroke Research Institute, Victoria, Australia

This book will be very useful for general practitioners, nurses and other members of the primary health care team in helping stroke victims negotiate their journey through their daily lives and the health system. I recommend it highly.

Ngaire Kerse, PhD, FRNZCGP
Associate Professor
Department of General Practice and Primary Health Care
The University of Auckland, New Zealand

Whether you are a stroke person, family, carer, or health professional, you will get a lot of practical information and help from this book.

Dr Harry McNaughton, PhD, FRACP, FAFRM
Honorary Medical Director
The Stroke Foundation of New Zealand

WHEN LIGHTNING STRIKES

An Illustrated Guide to Stroke
Prevention and Recovery

DR VALERY FEIGIN
MD, PhD

Senior Research Fellow, Clinical Trials Research Unit,
The University of Auckland, New Zealand

Endorsed by
The Stroke Foundation of New Zealand
The National Stroke Foundation of Australia

HarperCollins*Publishers*

To my parents and my family

National Library of New Zealand Cataloguing-in-Publication Data

Feigin, Valery L.
When lightning strikes : an illustrated guide to stroke prevention
and recovery / Valery Feigin.
Includes index.
ISBN 1-86950-535-2
1. Cerebrovascular disease—Popular works. I. Title.
616.81—dc 22

First published 2004
HarperCollins*Publishers* (New Zealand) Limited
P.O. Box 1, Auckland

ISBN 1 86950 535 2

Cover design by Judi Rowe
Internal text design and typesetting by Judi Rowe

Printed in China through Phoenix Offset, on 128 gsm matt art

Contents

Acknowledgments

In the preparation of this book I have used some scientific content from my previous handbooks and guidelines for doctors, including *Handbook of Stroke* and *Cerebrovascular Disease in Clinical Practice* (D.O. Wiebers, V.L. Feigin, R.D. Brown Jr; Lippincott-Raven Publishers, Philadelphia, 1997; Little, Brown and Company, Boston, 1997). I greatly appreciate the permission of the Mayo Clinic (Rochester, Minnesota, USA) to reuse some of the pictures from these handbooks. I am deeply indebted to my friends and colleagues at Middlemore Hospital and the Clinical Trials Research Unit of the University of Auckland, New Zealand, for a very supportive environment that encouraged me to write this book.

In particular, I would like to thank Professor David O. Wiebers (Mayo Clinic, Rochester, Minnesota, USA), Professor Geoffrey Donnan (National Stroke Research Institute, Victoria, Australia), Professor Graeme Hankey (Royal Perth Hospital, Australia), Professor Vladimir Hachinski (University of Western Ontario, London, Canada), Professor Charles Wolfe (Guy's and St Thomas' Hospital, London, UK), Dr Harry McNaughton (Medical Research Institute of New Zealand, Honorary Medical Director, the Stroke Foundation of New Zealand), Dr Ngaire Kerse (Associate Professor, Department of General Practice and Primary Health Care, the University of Auckland, New Zealand), Dr Anthony Rodgers, Dr Carlene Lawes, Dr Cliona Ni Mhurchu, Judy Murphy, Sheila Fisher, Mary Cosson (Clinical Trials Research Unit, the University of Auckland, New Zealand), Dr Alan Barber (Auckland Hospital, the University of Auckland, New Zealand), Judith Halliday (Ambassador, National Stroke Foundation of Australia) and Anne Liewelyn (the Stroke Foundation of New Zealand) for reviewing the first drafts of the manuscript. I express my profound gratitude to the dedicated team of specialists at the stroke unit and rehabilitation services of Middlemore Hospital, Auckland, New Zealand, including Dr Yogini Ratnasabapathy, Helen Walters, Felicity Stedman, Mark Harris, Caroline Berg, Vanessa Wiig and Maude Pomare-Hamlin, who provided extensive reviews and valuable commentaries on the manuscript. I am also enormously grateful to Dr Matthew Parsons (the University of Auckland, New Zealand), Annabel Grant and John Parsons (Waitemata District Health Board, Auckland, New Zealand) and Rochelle Bregmen (Auckland District Health Board, New Zealand) for their valuable comments regarding rehabilitation. I thank Dr Graeme Anderson for providing CT scans of the brain, and Mark Harris, Felicity Stedman, Caroline Berg (Middlemore Hospital), James Arthur Ellis and Lee-Yan Marquez (graphic artists) and Bill and Marion Steele for helping with the pictures. The photo on page 56 is used with permission of ResMed Limited, who own the copyright for the image. I also greatly appreciate the generous support of the Stroke Foundation of New Zealand in providing me with valuable suggestions and some of the illustrations. Finally, I would like to thank my wife, Tatiana Feigin, for her help, patience and support at every stage in the production of this book.

Foreword

Strokes impose an enormous burden on the patients themselves, their families and carers and on the community. Every year about 0.2 per cent of the population has a stroke, of whom nearly a third die over the next 12 months, a third remain permanently disabled (often requiring assistance from a carer) and a third regain their independence. Stroke survivors have an increased risk of another stroke or of a heart attack. Indeed, many fear another stroke because they regard a disabling stroke as a fate worse than death.

Strokes present an enormous challenge to the community because the number of people affected by them is likely to increase considerably in the near future. The risk of having a stroke increases with age, and our population is progressively ageing (we are surviving longer and the post World War II 'baby boomers' are now entering their fifties and sixties).

The two main strategies to reduce the burden are:

- to *prevent* first strokes in the general population and recurrent strokes among stroke survivors by recognising and controlling the risk factors that cause them
- to *treat* patients as soon as they do have a stroke to optimise their chances of surviving free from disabilities.

During the past decade there have been several advances in the treatment and rehabilitation of stroke patients, with an improvement in the number of people surviving free of dependency, but the greatest potential advances have been, and are likely to continue to be, in stroke prevention.

There have been public health campaigns aimed at educating the general population about the increased risk of a stroke caused by high blood pressure, smoking, diabetes and atrial fibrillation (irregular heartbeat). Lowering the incidence of these risk factors with simple lifestyle modifications can have a substantial impact on preventing strokes in the community.

People are encouraged to have their diet, lifestyle, heart rate, blood pressure, blood cholesterol and blood sugar checked, controlled (if necessary) and monitored in the same way that they would have any other valuable asset, such as a car, assessed and 'serviced' regularly.

For those who are assessed by their doctor to be at an increased likelihood of a stroke, the 'high risk' approach to prevention involves treatment with effective and appropriate medical and surgical interventions, some of which are costly and even slightly risky themselves.

In this marvellous book, Professor Valery Feigin provides a comprehensive and cutting edge, yet succinct, overview of all of these issues, as well as an informed and balanced insight into the causes and consequences of strokes and the interventions that can safely and effectively prevent them or optimise a patient's chances of surviving free from disabilities. Professor Feigin translates his vast experience and thorough knowledge of the medical literature into a light, easy-to-use text that's punctuated by superb illustrations, case reports and appendices — you should check your own risk of stroke (page 40) and try out the diet recommendations and recipes.

This book is written for the general public and accordingly the language is simple and clear throughout, and supplemented by a generous glossary. This is one of the very few books in which authoritative, up-to-date and useful medical information about strokes is distilled into a form that will be easily understood and made use of by the general public, particularly stroke survivors and their families and carers.

Graeme J. Hankey, MBBS, MD, FRCP, FRCP (Edin), FRACP
Consultant Neurologist and Head of Stroke Unit,
Royal Perth Hospital, Perth
Clinical Professor, School of Medicine and Pharmacology,
The University of Western Australia, Australia

'Life isn't an active force —
it's we who make what we will of it'
HENRY HANDEL RICHARDSON

Introduction

Stroke is the number one disabler and number two killer in the world. It has become a worldwide health problem of increasing importance, with two-thirds of strokes now occurring in the developing countries. Globally, approximately 80 million people are suffering from the results of a stroke at any given time. There are approximately 13 million new stroke victims each year, of which approximately 4.4 million die within 12 months. There are some 250 million direct family members of those survivors. During the course of their lives, about four out of five families will have someone affected by a stroke.

Stroke is one of the most destructive brain disorders with severe consequences, including enormous psychological, physical and financial pressure on the patients, their families and society. In fact many people are more fearful of being disabled by a stroke than of death itself. If there are no improvements in the current preventive methods, then the number of strokes and stroke victims will grow considerably over the next few decades.

A stroke used to be perceived as an unpredictable disorder that could happen to anyone, and that once it had happened there was nothing effective that could be done about it. However, recent scientific data have convincingly shown quite the opposite. The last decade has been a time of tremendous advancement in our understanding of stroke risk factors, prevention, treatment and rehabilitation. We now know that a stroke is highly predictable and can be prevented in up to 85 per cent of people. There are also effective treatments that can substantially improve the outcome of a stroke. In fact, approximately one third of stroke patients now recover fully, and this proportion could be even greater if adequate emergency and rehabilitation treatment was always received.

This book aims to provide a user-friendly, yet comprehensive, evidence-based illustrated guide for people without a special medical background who wish to prevent a stroke from happening or want to know how to deal with the consequences of stroke at a personal and family level. It also provides information about the most effective methods of stroke treatment.

1

Understanding
the brain

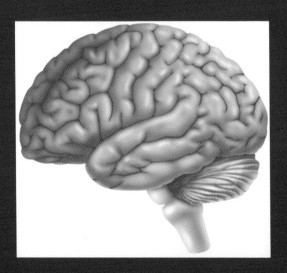

The basic anatomy of the brain and its blood supply

The brain is a vital organ. It's responsible for our individual mental and intellectual functions, such as thinking and memory. It controls our interactions with the outside world, for example, it interprets what our senses encounter and controls our voluntary movements. It also controls many of our automatic bodily functions. Up to 80 per cent of all human genes are used by the brain.

The brain consists of brain cells called neurons, supporting cells known as glial cells, cerebrospinal fluid and blood vessels. The arteries are the vessels that carry blood rich in oxygen and nutrients, such as glucose, to the brain. The veins are the vessels that take the depleted blood and waste products away. Everyone has a similar number of neurons — around 100 billion — but the number of connections between the different neurons varies. In an adult, the brain constitutes only about 2 per cent (approximately 1.4 kg) of the total body weight, but it consumes about 20 per cent of the oxygen and 50 per cent of the glucose in the arterial blood.

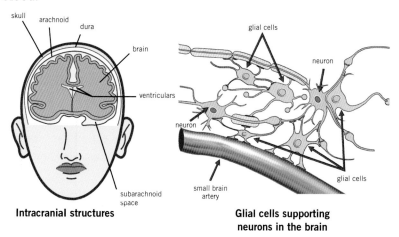

Intracranial structures

Glial cells supporting neurons in the brain

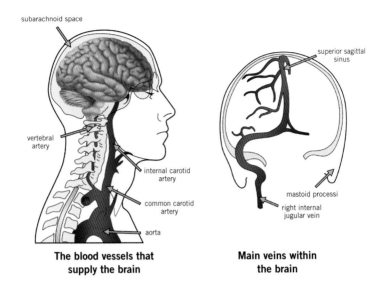

The blood vessels that supply the brain

Main veins within the brain

Significantly, the brain doesn't store oxygen and other nutrients, and so to function properly it depends entirely on a constant 24-hour supply from the circulating arterial blood. For normal functioning, the brain must receive approximately 1 litre of blood per minute, which is approximately 15 per cent of the total blood the heart pumps out when at rest. No other organ in the body consistently receives such an intensive blood supply.

The brain is supplied with arterial blood through a pair of major circulatory systems. The first consists of two arteries, called the carotid arteries, which supply blood to the front parts of the brain. This is known as the *anterior cerebral artery circulation*. The second is the vertebrobasilar system, which supplies the back of the brain. It's called the *posterior cerebral artery circulation*. The two systems are connected by blood vessels.

The neurons are the most sensitive of all the body's cells to a lack of oxygen in the blood. Just 7–10 seconds of interruption to the arterial blood supply to the brain can result in irreversible damage (neuron death) to the affected part of the brain. However, there are some mechanisms that can, to some extent, prevent brain damage and facilitate recovery. Unlike any other organ, the brain has its own system of auto-regulation, which ensures the consistency of the blood circulation within certain physiological limits. If the conditions exceed these limits, the auto-regulation system fails, resulting in a stroke.

The basics of brain functioning

Different parts of the brain control different physical, emotional and behavioural functions. The two brain hemispheres are not exactly symmetrical, anatomically or functionally. However, they're connected anatomically and are functionally interrelated. In right-handed people and about half of left-handed people, the left side of the brain controls the ability to understand and produce language and is more related to 'mathematical' or 'logical' thinking, while the right side of the brain controls spatial orientation and is more related to

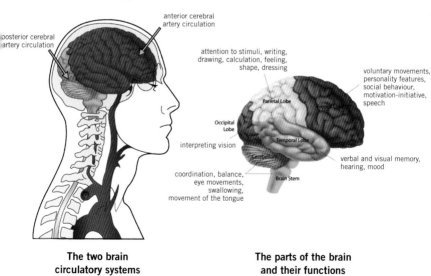

posterior cerebral
artery circulation

anterior cerebral
artery circulation

attention to stimuli, writing,
drawing, calculation, feeling,
shape, dressing

voluntary movements,
personality features,
social behaviour,
motivation-initiative,
speech

Parietal Lobe

Occipital
Lobe

interpreting vision

Temporal Lobe

Cerebellum

coordination, balance,
eye movements,
swallowing,
movement of the tongue

Brain Stem

verbal and visual memory,
hearing, mood

**The two brain
circulatory systems**

**The parts of the brain
and their functions**

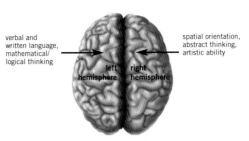

verbal and
written language,
mathematical/
logical thinking

spatial orientation,
abstract thinking,
artistic ability

left
hemisphere

right
hemisphere

The two hemispheres of the brain

abstract thinking and imaginary and artistic abilities. It's the other way round for the rest of the population.

The anterior (or front) parts of the brain, which receive blood from the anterior cerebral artery circulation, control the opposite sides of the body from where they're located. If, for example, brain damage occurs in the right anterior circulation area, it may affect the movements and senses on the left side of the body, and vice versa.

If brain damage occurs in the posterior parts of the brain, which receive blood from the posterior cerebral circulation, it may affect both sides of the body. There could, for example, be weakness on one side of the body and numbness on the other side. There could also be problems with swallowing, breathing, language, balance or coordination, or abnormal head-and-upper-body movements.

(See Appendix 1 for more information about the relationship between the location of stroke damage and the possible symptoms.)

Brain plasticity

The brain is a very adaptable organ. Recent studies show that brain growth and nerve-cell change are not limited to childhood as previously thought. Although dead neurons don't regenerate, the adaptive ability, or plasticity, of the human brain is amazing, especially in young people. There is evidence that in some situations parts of the brain can take over lost functions from other damaged parts. In other words, parts of the brain somehow learn new abilities. This may be the most important mechanism involved in stroke recovery.

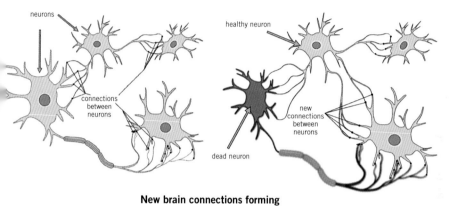

neurons

connections between neurons

healthy neuron

new connections between neurons

dead neuron

New brain connections forming

KEY INFORMATION

■ The brain is a unique organ that determines our mental functions and controls our behaviour and other bodily functions.

■ The brain is completely dependent on its blood supply. An interruption of about 7–10 seconds can result in irreversible damage to the affected part of the brain.

■ The blood supply to the brain is provided by two systems of arteries: the carotid arteries (anterior cerebral artery circulation) and the vertebral arteries (posterior cerebral artery circulation).

■ The brain can repair itself to some extent, but its adaptive ability (plasticity) isn't fully understood.

2

Understanding strokes

What is a stroke and what is a TIA?

A stroke is an acute vascular injury of the brain. This means that it's a sudden, severe injury to the brain's blood vessels. The injury can be caused by a blood-clot blockage, by narrowing of the blood vessels (clogging), by both a blockage and narrowing, or by a rupture of the blood vessels. All these things result in a lack of adequate blood supply. Depending on the site and size of the damage, a stroke may or may not produce symptoms (a symptomless stroke is called a silent stroke).

The symptoms of a stroke can be physical, psychological and/or behavioural. The most typical physical symptoms include paralysis, weakness (sometime described by patients as clumsiness), a loss of sensation in the face, arm or leg on one side of the body, difficulty talking and/or understanding (without hearing problems), difficulty swallowing and a partial loss of vision on one side. A person is said to have had a

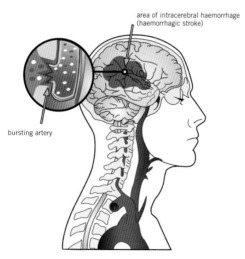

area of intracerebral haemorrhage
(haemorrhagic stroke)

bursting artery

An intracerebral haemorrhage

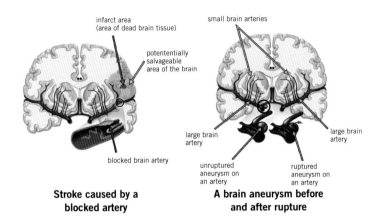

Stroke caused by a blocked artery

A brain aneurysm before and after rupture

stroke if one or any combination of these symptoms lasts 24 hours or longer. However, a person is said to have had a *transient ischaemic attack* (TIA) if all the symptoms disappear within 24 hours.

A TIA, also called a *mini* or *minor stroke*, is a major risk factor for an ischaemic stroke (a stroke caused by a blockage or narrowing of one or more arteries leading to the brain). This means that if a person has a TIA they're at a high risk of having an ischaemic stroke and should see a doctor immediately. The symptoms usually come on quickly and last 10 seconds to 15 minutes. Occasionally they can last as long as 24 hours. In a typical TIA, the symptoms usually reach maximum intensity within 2 minutes, often within a few seconds. It used to be thought that a TIA left no permanent brain-tissue damage but modern diagnostic investigations show that in up to 50 per cent of people there's some damage, usually brain infarction (tissue death) or sometimes a small haemorrhage (see pages 14–16 for details).

Clinically, a symptomless stroke causes no symptoms and can only be detected by using special neuroimaging techniques, such as *computerised tomography* (CT) or *magnetic resonance tomography* (MRT) of the head. However, if a symptomless stroke is detected, it shouldn't be left without medical attention because it may eventually lead to devastating complications, including symptomatic strokes, progressive dementia and behavioural disorders.

> ### EXAMPLE OF A TYPICAL STROKE-CLINIC PATIENT
>
> A 55-year-old woman complained of episodes of unprovoked clumsiness or weakness in her right hand, which had started about a month earlier. Initially, each episode lasted for a few seconds and completely disappeared, usually spontaneously, but sometimes after rubbing her hand. She was a smoker but otherwise generally healthy. She attributed the episodes to her intensive work and tiredness, and didn't initially seek medical attention. However, she had noticed that the episodes were starting to last longer, and the most recent episode didn't completely resolve itself for about 2 days. Clinical examination confirmed that the woman had suffered from a minor ischaemic stroke in the left anterior cerebral artery circulation caused by narrowing (stenosis) of her left carotid artery in the neck.

What are the warning signs and symptoms of a stroke or TIA?

Although two-thirds of strokes occur without any warning, approximately one third do have warning signs, including TIAs. Call an ambulance immediately if you or someone else has any of the following symptoms (especially if they come on suddenly):

- loss of strength (or development of clumsiness) in some part of the body, especially on one side, including the face, arm or leg
- numbness (sensory loss) or other unusual sensations in some part of the body, especially if they're one sided

Lesion on the right thalamus

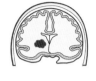
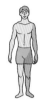

weakness and sensory loss on the left side of the body

Lesion on the right half of the brain stem

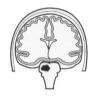

weakness and sensory loss on the left side of the body and the right side of the face

- complete or partial loss of vision on one side
- an inability to speak properly or to understand language
- loss of balance, unsteadiness or an unexplained fall
- any other kind of transient spell, such as vertigo, dizziness, swallowing difficulties, acute confusion or memory disturbances

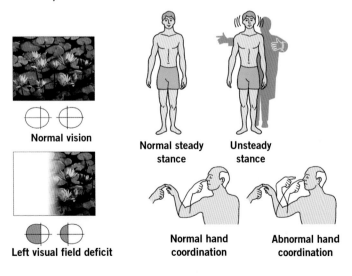

Normal vision

Normal steady stance

Unsteady stance

Left visual field deficit

Normal hand coordination

Abnormal hand coordination

■ a headache that's unusually severe, begins abruptly or is of unusual character, including an unexplained change in the pattern of headaches

■ unexplained alterations of consciousness or convulsions.

These warning signs may occur alone or in any combination. They may last a few seconds (a typical TIA) or up to 24 hours (an atypical, severe TIA), and could happen only once during a day or be repeated. By definition, during the first 24 hours after the symptoms appear it's impossible to know for sure if they're caused by a stroke or a TIA. Even if it's a TIA, the symptoms can indicate a hidden problem with the blood flow in the brain, which, if ignored, could result in a stroke, so don't wait to seek medical help.

What if I suspect it's a stroke?

If you suspect it's a stroke (see above for warning signs), call an ambulance as soon as possible by dialling:

■ 111 in New Zealand
■ 000 in Australia
■ 999 in the UK
■ 911 in the USA and Canada.

Then follow these emergency procedures.

■ If the person is unconscious, check their breathing and pulse and loosen any restrictive clothing that could cause breathing difficulties. If the person has collapsed indoors, place them on a bed or sofa. Try to lie them on their side with their head slightly elevated (10–30 degrees). Minimise any bending in their neck, and make sure that their airways are clear of any saliva or vomit. Remove any dentures from their mouth. (Never lay an unconscious person on their back as it can lead to choking or blocking of the airways by the tongue.)

- If the patient vomits or has difficulty breathing, try to keep them lying on their side (preferably with less time on left side) with their head slightly raised.
- If the person has a fit (seizure), try to remove any objects they could hit while convulsing. Don't restrain the person in any way or put your fingers or hard objects (such as a spoon) in their mouth because your fingers could be bitten or the person's teeth could be broken.
- Don't give the affected person anything to eat or drink because of the risk of choking or of breathing food or liquid into the lungs.
- If there's obvious weakness in an arm or leg, help support that limb and avoid pulling on it when moving the person.

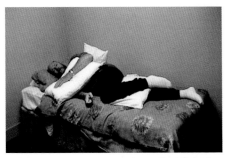

The correct way to support a patient in bed

What is an ischaemic stroke?

Up to 85 per cent of strokes are caused by either:
— a blockage from a blood clot
— narrowing (clogging) of an artery or arteries leading to the brain, or
— emboli (debris) breaking away from the heart or an extracranial artery (an artery outside the cranium) causing a blockage in one or a few of the intracranial arteries (arteries within the brain).
This is called brain infarction or an ischaemic stroke. In

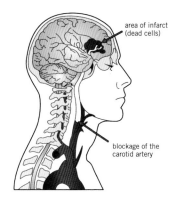

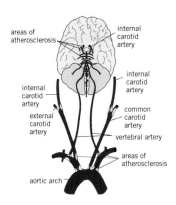

Stroke caused by a blood clot   **Atherosclerosis**

people over 65 years, the blockage or narrowing can be caused by atherosclerosis (hardening of arteries). This is the case with as many as two-thirds of ischaemic stroke patients. Embolisms tend to occur most often in people with substantial heart disease (such as rapid irregular heartbeats, heart-valve disease, etc.; see pages 21–23). On average, a quarter of ischaemic strokes are caused by an embolism, usually from the heart (cardioembolic strokes). Clots from the heart most commonly arise from irregular heartbeats (e.g. atrial fibrillation), abnormal heart valves (including artificial valves and damaged valves from rheumatic heart disease), infections inside the heart (known as endocarditis) and heart surgery.

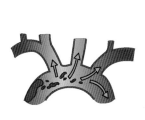

Emboli from the internal carotid artery and aorta

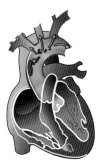

Heart with flying emboli

Other causes such as blood disorders, inflammation and infection are responsible for about 5–10 per cent of ischaemic strokes, and are the most common causes in young people. However, the exact cause of some ischaemic strokes remains undetermined even after extensive investigations.

Most ischaemic strokes occur in the brain hemispheres, though some occur in the cerebellum or the brain stem. Some ischaemic strokes in the hemispheres seem minor (about 20 per cent of all ischaemic strokes); they're either asymptomatic (this happens in about a third of older people) or cause only clumsiness, minor weakness (usually just in one arm) or memory problems. However, multiple and repeated minor strokes can lead to severe disability, cognitive decline and dementia.

What is a haemorrhagic stroke?

A haemorrhagic stroke is caused by bleeding into the brain tissue (called an intracerebral haemorrhage or intracerebral haematoma) or into the subarachnoid space, the narrow space between the brain surface and the layer of tissue that covers the brain (called a subarachnoid haemorrhage). These are the most lethal types of stroke, but they make up a relatively small proportion of total strokes: 10–15 per cent for intracerebral haemorrhages and approximately 5 per cent for subarachnoid haemorrhages.

Bleeding from an intracranial artery is usually caused by an aneurysm (dilated artery) that ruptures or because of some disease.

Diseases that make the artery walls thin and brittle are the most common causes of intracerebral haemorrhages. Such diseases include hypertension (elevated blood pressure) or amyloid angiopathy (where protein is deposited in the walls of small arteries in the brain). When someone has an intracerebral haemorrhage, blood is forced into the brain tissue,

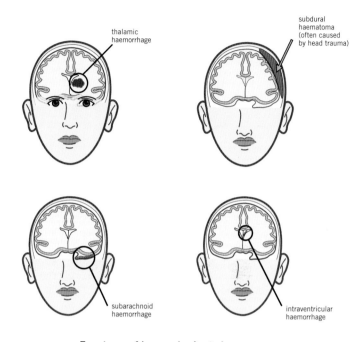

Four types of haemorrhagic stroke

damaging neurons (brain cells) so that the affected part of the brain can't function properly.

Rupture of an aneurysm is the most common cause of subarachnoid haemorrhages. In a subarachnoid haemorrhage, blood is forced into the subarachnoid space surrounding the brain. The brain tissue isn't usually affected at first, but can be at later stages.

Sometimes, a headache can be the only symptom of a subarachnoid haemorrhage, but if it's ignored it can lead to catastrophic consequences. A typical subarachnoid haemorrhage headache comes on suddenly, is severe and has no apparent cause. Patients describe it as 'like being hit over the head with a hammer', 'the worst headache of my life' or 'like someone's trying to kick their way out of the top of my head'.

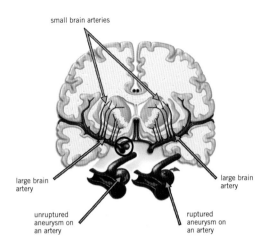

small brain arteries

large brain
artery

large brain
artery

unruptured
aneurysm on
an artery

ruptured
aneurysm on
an artery

An aneurysm before and after rupture

It's often accompanied by vomiting, a stiff neck or a temporary loss of consciousness. If you or anyone else has these symptoms, call an ambulance straight away.

Up to 30 per cent of all subarachnoid haemorrhages, however, have different symptoms to those described above; and a small subarachnoid haemorrhage, especially in an older person, may not necessarily result in a very severe headache or have a catastrophic onset. Because of this, any headache that comes on abruptly should be a prompt to seek immediate medical attention.

KEY INFORMATION

- There are several types of stroke: ischaemic stroke, intracerebral haemorrhage and subarachnoid haemorrhage. They differ in their causes and in the damage done to the brain.
- A transient ischaemic attack (TIA) is a minor stroke but if left untreated it can lead to a major stroke.
- The most typical warning signs of a stroke are sudden loss of strength, numbness or visual loss on one side of the body, or sudden speech, swallowing or balancing difficulties.
- A sudden severe headache may be the only warning symptom of a subarachnoid haemorrhage.
- Anyone with the warning symptoms of a stroke (even a suspected stroke) should seek immediate medical attention.

3

Understanding stroke risk factors

Most strokes result from a combination of medical causes (such as elevated blood pressure) and behavioural causes (such as smoking). These causes are called 'risk factors'.

Some risk factors can be controlled or eradicated completely either by medical means, such as taking certain medications, or by non-medical means, such as a change in lifestyle. These are called modifiable risk factors. It's thought that up to 85 per cent of all strokes can be prevented by controlling the modifiable risk factors.

There are some risk factors, however, that can't be changed. The non-modifiable risk factors include ageing, genetic predisposition and ethnicity.

The medical risk factors include:

- hypertension (high blood pressure)
- high levels of fatty substances such as cholesterol in the blood
- atherosclerosis (hardening of arteries)
- various heart disorders, including atrial fibrillation (e.g. an irregular heartbeat), diabetes and an unruptured intracranial aneurysm
- a family history of stroke and other genetic markers
- migraines.

Many of these risk factors are interrelated and may aggravate one another. For example, people with elevated blood pressure tend to suffer more often from heart disease and atherosclerosis; and diabetes promotes atherosclerosis and elevated blood pressure. The risk of having a stroke increases with a combination of the risk factors. Most risk factors, however, are avoidable or can be efficiently controlled.

Behavioural risk factors are ones that result from a person's behaviour or lifestyle. The most important ones are smoking (active and passive), an unhealthy diet, excess alcohol consumption, a sedentary lifestyle, snoring and sleep apnoea, oral contraceptives, recreational drugs (such as heroin, amphetamines, cocaine and marijuana) and being overweight.

Hypertension

An adult's blood pressure is categorised as normal if their systolic blood pressure (the pressure when the heart is contracting) is below 120 mm Hg and their diastolic blood pressure (the pressure when the heart is filling) is below 80 mm Hg, regardless of their age or sex. This is often described as 120/80 mg Hg.

High blood pressure is called hypertension. The increased risk of a stroke and other cardiovascular disease begins at 115/75 mm Hg and doubles with each increment of 20/10 mm Hg. People who have definite hypertension (a systolic blood pressure greater than or equal to 140 mm Hg or a diastolic blood pressure greater than or equal to 90 mm Hg) have a seven times higher risk of a stroke than those with normal or low blood pressure. For people aged over 50, a high systolic blood pressure (140 mm Hg or higher) is considered a greater risk factor for a stroke and other cardiovascular disease than a high diastolic blood pressure. However, blood pressure tends to increase with age, and people who have normal blood pressure at 55 have almost a two-fold risk for developing hypertension compared with younger people.

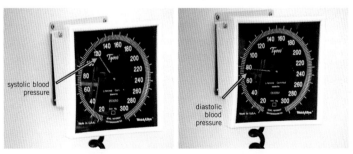

Systolic and diastolic blood pressure readings

An elevated blood pressure gradually damages the blood-vessel walls by hardening the arteries and promoting the formation of blood clots and aneurysms, all of which can lead to a stroke, especially in people over 45. Studies show that somewhere between a third and almost a half of all people over 45 suffer from hypertension. One of the main problems with hypertension is that it has no symptoms in the early stages. It can cause chronic or occasional headaches in some people, but up to 30 per cent of people with the condition are unaware they have it, and even less do anything to control it. Because of this it is sometimes called a 'silent killer'. That's why, after reaching 40, it's important to have your blood pressure checked regularly — at least once a year until the age of 55 and twice a year after that. In situations where there's a family history of stroke, hypertension or angina or where there are other risk factors present such as smoking or heart disease, it's advisable to have your blood pressure checked regularly at an even earlier age, at 30, say.

Heart disease

People with heart problems, such as angina, atrial fibrillation, heart failure, valve disorders, artificial valves and congenital heart defects, are at an increased risk of having a stroke. Blood

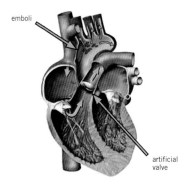

emboli

artificial valve

Emboli resulting from a heart-valve disorder

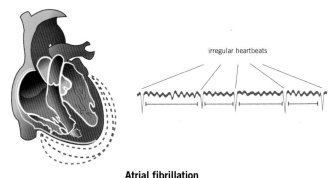

Atrial fibrillation

clots, known as emboli, sometimes form in the heart as a result of heart-valve disorders, irregular heartbeat rhythms or after a heart attack and can break loose and travel to the brain or other parts of the body. Once in the brain, a clot can block an artery and cause an ischaemic stroke.

One of the most significant risk factors for a stroke is atrial fibrillation (AF). AF is classified as a type of irregular heartbeat where the left atrium of the heart beats rapidly and unpredictably. Some people with paroxysmal AF (AF that comes on occasionally) can feel a 'pounding' sensation or

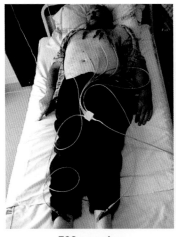

ECG procedure

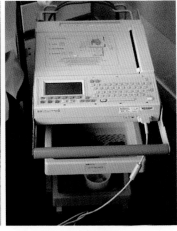

ECG machine

'fluttering heartbeats' or 'missing heartbeats', known as heart palpitations. In other people, the only symptom of AF is occasional dizziness, faintness or light-headedness, or various degrees of chest pain. The only reliable method of diagnosing the condition is electrocardiography (see page 74). Untreated AF increases the risk of stroke by four to seven times, and can lead to other cardiovascular complications, including a potentially fatal embolism in the pulmonary artery and heart failure.

Atherosclerosis

Atherosclerosis (hardening of the arteries) is one of the leading causes of strokes, especially ischaemic strokes and TIAs. In about 20–30 per cent of patients who've had an ischaemic stroke or TIA, the primary cause is narrowing of the carotid artery in the neck.

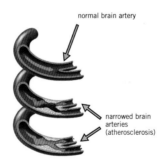

normal brain artery

narrowed brain arteries (atherosclerosis)

Atherosclerosis

High cholesterol levels

Although lipids (fatty substances) are integral components of our bodies, a high level of blood lipids (especially cholesterol and triglycerides) increases the risk of atherosclerosis and coronary heart disease. It's also associated with an approximately 20 per cent increased risk of an ischaemic stroke or a TIA.

There are two main types of cholesterol: 'bad' cholesterol (cholesterol carried by low-density and very-low-density lipoproteins) and 'good' cholesterol (cholesterol carried by high-density lipoproteins).

'Bad' cholesterol sticks to artery walls and contributes to the development of arterial plaques, which lead to athero-sclerosis (artery hardening) and stenosis (narrowing), and contribute to the formation of blood clots, thus increasing the risk of an ischaemic stroke or a TIA.

'Good' cholesterol carries 'bad' cholesterol away from the arteries, thus reducing the risk of atherosclerosis and an ischaemic stroke or TIA. The desirable level of 'good' choles-terol is 40 mg/dL (1.04 mmol/L) or above, whereas a person's levels of 'bad' cholesterol and total cholesterol should ideally be less than 100 mg/dL (2.59 mmol/L) and 200 mg/dL (5.18 mmol/L), respectively.

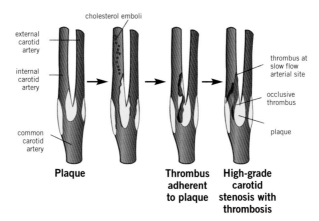

cholesterol emboli

external carotid artery

internal carotid artery

common carotid artery

thrombus at slow flow arterial site

occlusive thrombus

plaque

Plaque   **Thrombus adherent to plaque**   **High-grade carotid stenosis with thrombosis**

Transient ischaemic attack (TIA)

Approximately two out of every hundred adults will have at least one transient ischaemic attack (TIA) in their lifetime. If not treated adequately, about one tenth of these patients will go on to have a stroke (usually an ischaemic stroke) within

3 months of the first attack, and about one third will have a stroke within five years of the first attack. The probability of having a stroke increases by approximately 1.5 fold for each 10 years of increasing age and is higher in those who have multiple TIAs of increasing frequency.

Diabetes

Diabetes mellitus is a common disorder affecting approximately 1 in 30 adults. Having the disease, however, doubles the chance of having a stroke because it leads to changes in the vascular system (the blood vessels and heart) and promotes atherosclerosis. Common symptoms of diabetes include excessive and frequent urination, excessive thirst, unexplained tiredness and lack of energy and a tendency to get infections, especially of the skin. There are two types of diabetes: type I and type II. Type I usually starts at a young age and requires regular injections of insulin (insulin-dependent diabetes mellitus). Type II mainly affects people over 40 and in the initial stages can usually be controlled with tablets and dietary modifications.

Gender and ageing

Men younger than 65 are at an approximately 20 per cent higher risk of having an ischaemic stroke or intracerebral haemorrhage than women. Women of any age, however, have about a 50 per cent higher risk of a subarachnoid haemorrhage. Women are also three times more likely than men to develop unruptured intracranial aneurysms. These gender differences are less prominent in young adults, where strokes affect men and women almost equally.

The risk of having a stroke increases from the age of 45. After reaching 50, every subsequent 3 years of ageing is associated with an increased stroke risk of between 11 and 20 per cent, with the increase going up with age. People over 65 have the highest risk, but up to 25 per cent of all strokes occur in adults younger than this, and up to 4 per cent occur in people aged between 15 and 40.

Strokes are uncommon in children younger than 15, but when they do occur it's usually the result of congenital heart disease, blood-vessel malformations, head or neck trauma, migraine or a blood disease.

Family history and genetics

Heredity conditions are very rarely direct causes of a stroke. However, genes do play a large role in some stroke risk factors, such as hypertension, heart disease, diabetes and vascular malformations. A family history of stroke, especially if two or more family members have had a stroke younger than 65, increases the chance of having a stroke. There are also some rare genetic disorders that increase the risk of having a stroke, including polycystic kidney disease, Ehlers-Danlos syndrome type IV, neurofibromatosis, type I Marfans syndrome, a generic mutation in factor V Leiden, and inherited deficiencies in factors called protein C and S.

It's also known that strokes (especially haemorrhagic strokes) are more common amongst people of African, Asian, Afro-Caribbean, Maori and Pacific island origin than people of European origin. For example, strokes affect Maori and Pacific island people 10–15 years earlier than Europeans. The reasons for this are not clear but there's a higher incidence of hypertension, diabetes and other risk factors in these populations. However, it should be stressed that most of these risk factors are modifiable and can potentially be managed to reduce the risk.

Genetic factors are particularly important with regard to subarachnoid haemorrhages, possibly accounting for 7 per cent of the total cases and up to 20 per cent in young people. First-degree relatives (children) of people who've had a subarachnoid haemorrhage have a 2–5 per cent increase in their risk of having a subarachnoid haemorrhage themselves.

Unruptured intracranial aneurysms

An aneurysm is a weak spot in an artery wall that balloons out. It's a relatively common abnormality — on the average, 2–5 per cent of adults have a brain aneurysm at some point in their lives. However, aneurysms burst in only 2 out of every 10,000 people aged 55 years or older. Therefore if an unruptured intracranial aneurysm is detected during a brain scan it doesn't necessarily mean it will burst. Whether it happens or not may depend on several factors, including the presence of clinical symptoms, the size of the aneurysm, polycystic kidney disease, a family history of subarachnoid haemorrhages and other associated risk factors, especially smoking and hypertension.

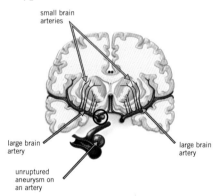

An unruptured aneurysm

It's critically important that anyone with a detected unruptured aneurysm is seen regularly by a neurosurgeon or neurologist, who will help to control the risk factors and advise on the most appropriate time for aneurysm surgery. The most common form of surgery is coiling or clipping to obliterate the aneurysm.

The most important modifiable risk factors for the growth of intracranial aneurysms and possibly for their rupture are active smoking and hypertension. Fortunately, the risk of having a subarachnoid haemorrhage diminishes rapidly after giving up smoking, and people who give up active smoking for 15 years are at the same risk of aneurysm rupture as people who've never smoked.

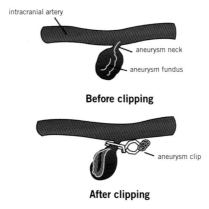

Before clipping

After clipping

Migraines

A migraine is a special form of headache that should be diagnosed by a doctor. Migraines, especially when preceded by a sensation of flashing lights (aura), are a stroke risk factor for both men and women, particularly women under 50 who also smoke and take oral contraceptives. However, the stroke risk for migraine sufferers diminishes with age.

Other medical problems

A number of other medical conditions may contribute to the risk of having a stroke. These include various disorders of the blood, such as sickle-cell disease and other blood clotting abnormalities, and the presence anti-phospholipid antibodies. These medical conditions are relatively rare causes of strokes and are most common in patients younger than 45 years.

Smoking

Smoking quadruples the risk of having a stroke. This applies to all types of tobacco smoking (cigarettes, pipes or cigars) and for all types of stroke, especially subarachnoid haemorrhages and ischaemic strokes. Smoking constricts and hardens the arteries throughout the body (including those in the brain, heart and legs), and so promotes atherosclerosis, reduces the blood flow and makes the blood more likely to clot. It also promotes the formation and growth of intracranial aneurysms.

Modern studies show that the risk of having a stroke is approximately 20 per cent higher for female smokers than it is for male smokers and that women are generally more sensitive to the hazardous effects of smoking. Even passive smoking (the second-hand inhalation of smoke) increases the chances of having a stroke by almost 80 per cent. The risk of a stroke is proportional to the amount and duration of smoke inhalation. Those who smoke 20 or more cigarettes a day have almost twice the risk of those who smoke less. The longer the smoking continues the greater the risk of having a stroke.

Unhealthy diet

To maintain their weight, the average adult needs a daily food intake of approximately 30–35 kcal for every kilogram of body weight. For older people these requirements may be less, especially if they're not physically active.

Food is our only source of energy, but different types of food have different calorie contents. On average:

- fats (such as regular butter, cooking oil, meat fat and margarine) provide 9 kcal/g
- proteins (such as meats and other animal products including milk and dairy foods, beans and other pulses) provide 4 kcal/g

- carbohydrates (such as breads, cereals, fruits and vegetables) provide 4 kcal/g
- alcohol provides 7 kcal/g.

If a person consumes more calories than they use up in everyday activity, the excess is transformed into fat, which accumulates in the body.

An unhealthy, poorly balanced diet (for example, a diet high in saturated fat, cholesterol or salt and low in fruit and vegetables) is one of the most significant stroke risk factors. Such a diet can cause and accelerate atherosclerosis (narrowing and hardening of arteries), hypertension, blood clots, diabetes and weight problems, all of which are known to be important stroke risk factors. Although there's no strong evidence that drinking coffee is associated with an increased risk of having a stroke, an excessive coffee intake (more than 6 cups of strong coffee a day) may pose a risk, especially in older people with hypertension, because it can lead to elevated blood pressure and cholesterol levels.

Alcohol excess

Although mild alcohol consumption (less than 30 grams per day for men and less than 15 grams for women — see Personal Stroke Risk chart on page 40) lowers stroke risk (especially of ischaemic stroke), regular drinking exceeding this level, binge drinking (drinking 75 grams of alcohol or more within a 24-hour period) and alcoholism all increase the blood pressure and so increase the risk of a stroke (especially a haemorrhagic stroke) by several times. To calculate how much alcohol you're consuming, it's important to know the amount of alcohol in each drink.

In Australia and New Zealand a 'standard drink' is one that contains 10 grams of alcohol, but different countries have different measures. A standard drink is 8 grams in the UK and 13.5 grams in Canada. In Australia, New Zealand

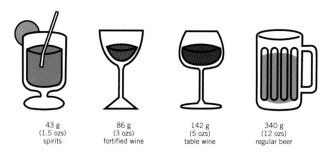

43 g
(1.5 ozs)
spirits

86 g
(3 ozs)
fortified wine

142 g
(5 ozs)
table wine

340 g
(12 ozs)
regular beer

Equivalents to one standard drink (10 g) of alcohol.

and the UK, it's recommended that the maximum number of standard drinks per week shouldn't exceed 14 for women and 21 drinks for men. It should be noted that lean people and older people are usually more sensitive to alcohol than younger people of normal weight.

It is important to remember that even mild alcohol consumption increases the blood pressure and should be avoided by people with hypertension. Also, some blood-pressure lowering drugs are incompatible with alcohol and can cause severe medical complications. Alcohol should be avoided completely by anyone who has epilepsy or a serious liver disorder or who is pregnant (especially during the first 3 months).

Physical inactivity

Physically inactive people (those who exercise for less than 30 minutes three times or less per week) have an almost 50 per cent greater risk of having a stroke than active people. Physical inactivity can lead to weight problems and increased blood pressure and is associated with diabetes, all of which are important stroke risk factors. Inactivity may also contribute to the early development of atherosclerosis and other cardiovascular complications, such as a heart attack.

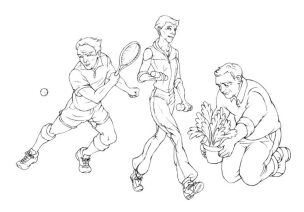

Find a physical activity that you enjoy.

Snoring and sleep apnoea

Snoring on its own isn't a stroke risk factor, however, if it's accompanied by sleep apnoea (regular periods of non-breathing that last longer than 10 seconds) there may be an increased likelihood of having a stroke during sleep. This is especially so for people with compromised heart function (e.g. congestive heart failure) or insufficient blood flow to the brain (e.g. through significant narrowing of major brain arteries or because of a previous stroke or TIA). Signs of sleep apnoea may include chronically disrupted sleep, waking in the night gasping for air, fatigue and sleepiness during the day.

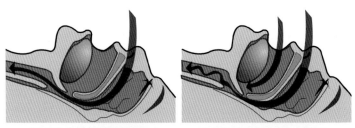

Normal air flow during sleep   **Snoring (obstructed airflow)**

Oral contraceptives

Most oral contraceptives contain both estrogen and progestogen; they're called combined oral contraceptives, and they can raise the blood pressure and make the blood stickier and more susceptible to forming clots. Combined oral contraceptives increase the risk of an ischaemic stroke, especially in women older than 30 who smoke.

Another type of oral contraceptive is the progestogen-only pill, also known as the mini-pill. Women using progestogen-only pills are at a lower risk of having a stroke. Former users of oral contraceptives who no longer take them have no excess stroke risk.

Hormone replacement therapy (HRT)

Hormone replacement therapy (HRT) is prescribed to some menopausal or post-menopausal women to increase the strength of their bones and to reduce the risk of colorectal cancer. However, there's evidence that HRT (especially a combination of estrogen with progestogen) increases the risk of a stroke by approximately 33 per cent, especially an ischaemic stroke. It also increases the risk of coronary heart disease and dementia.

Pregnancy

Strokes are uncommon among women of child-bearing age, although pregnancy has long been recognised as a factor that increases the risk of a stroke in young women. Haemorrhagic strokes cause 5–10 per cent of all maternal deaths that occur during pregnancy. Factors that increase the risk of a stroke in pregnant women include: increased maternal age, intracranial aneurysms and vascular malformations, rheumatic and other heart diseases causing valve abnormalities or cardiomyopathy (an enlarged heart with decreased heart-muscle functioning), inflammatory disorders of the arteries, blood disorders and hypertension. The risk of a stroke is also relatively high in the first 6 weeks following childbirth.

Stress and depression

Sometimes work, relationships, finances and other factors cause psychological stress, and it's not always possible to remove the cause. Although most stroke experts don't consider occasional episodes of stress a stroke risk factor, long-term stress can lead to elevated blood-pressure and cholesterol levels. A sudden emotional stress or shock, either positive or negative, when combined with other risk factors (e.g. severe atherosclerosis, heart disease or hypertension) may also trigger a stroke.

Depression can result from psychosocial stress (e.g. grief) or from biological dysfunction. Persistent untreated insomnia (insufficient or poor-quality sleep with a feeling of constant tiredness) is a strong risk factor for major depression. The most common symptoms of depression include: a depressed mood most of the day, a diminished interest or pleasure in all or almost all activities, a loss of appetite, excessive sleepiness or insomnia, chronic fatigue, feelings of worthlessness or excessive or inappropriate guilt nearly every day, a chronically diminished ability to think or concentrate and recurrent thoughts of death.

Depression almost doubles the risk of having a stroke. The exact mechanism for this isn't fully understood but there's evidence that depression can lead to hypertension, ischaemic heart disease and increased blood clotting, all factors known to be associated with the risk of a stroke.

Recreational drugs

Heroin, amphetamines, cocaine, phencyclidine, marijuana and other recreational drugs can all cause a stroke resulting from inflammation of the arteries and veins, a spasm of the arteries in the brain, heart dysfunction, increased blood clotting or a sudden increase in blood pressure.

Being overweight

The body mass index (BMI) is used to work out whether a person is overweight or obese. A person's BMI is calculated as their weight in kilograms divided by their height in metres squared. For example, if a person's weight is 98 kg and their height is 1.82 m, then their BMI is $98/1.82^2 = 29.6$ kg/m^2. You can also use a BMI table to work this out (see page 163).

For adults, a person is defined as overweight if they have a BMI exceeding 25. A BMI of 18.5 to 24.9 is considered a healthy weight, and a BMI of less than 18.5 is considered underweight. Being overweight increases the risk of a stroke by about 15 per cent by promoting hypertension, heart disease, type II diabetes and atherosclerosis. There's also some evidence that being underweight may increase the risk of having a subarachnoid haemorrhage.

Neck injuries

Neck injuries, including sudden and severe extension of the neck, neck rotation, intensive brain/neck radiation or pressure on an artery, can damage the vertebral or carotid arteries and cause a stroke, especially an ischaemic stroke in young adults. These types of injuries can occur in various circumstances, including improperly performed chiropractic manipulation of the neck.

Other risk factors

Low body temperatures in winter may increase the risk of a stroke by increasing blood pressure and promoting blood clotting, especially in older people and people with other stroke risk factors.

There's also some evidence that recent viral and bacterial infections may act with other factors to add a small increase in the risk of a stroke by increasing the clotting abilities of the blood.

KEY INFORMATION

- Strokes don't strike randomly but usually affect those who have stroke risk factors.
- The most important stroke risk factors are hypertension, smoking, atherosclerosis, heart disease, diabetes and an unhealthy diet.
- Different types of stroke are affected by different risk factors.

4

Estimating and managing your own risk of a stroke

The good thing about strokes is that they're highly preventable. In fact, up to 85 per cent of all strokes can be prevented. The key elements are:

- preventing risk factors from developing
- eliminating as many existing risk factors as possible
- diminishing exposure to any risk factors that can't be eliminated.

The best way to prevent or reduce risk factors is a healthy lifestyle, which means having a healthy diet, adequate physical activity and being emotionally balanced. To be as effective as possible, a healthy lifestyle should begin during childhood and continue throughout life.

There's also some evidence that a predisposition or resistance to many disorders, including strokes, may start as early as conception and continue to build up during pregnancy. While pregnant, especially at the early stages, such factors as smoking, drinking alcohol, stress and inadequate eating can all have adverse effects on the risk of a stroke and other cardiovascular disease in the unborn child's later life. On the other hand, avoiding these factors during pregnancy may reduce the risk of the child experiencing a stroke and many other chronic disorders when they're an adult themselves.

Stroke risk factors are discussed in the previous chapter, and can be divided into two groups: modifiable (factors that can be changed or altered) and non-modifiable (factors that can't be changed). The most important modifiable risk factors are: smoking, hypertension, atherosclerosis, heart disease, diabetes, unruptured intracranial aneurysms, alcohol excess, an unhealthy diet, being overweight, a sedentary lifestyle, chronic stress and depression. Non-modifiable risk factors include increasing age, male gender, particular ethnicity (people of African, Afro-Caribbean, Asian, Maori and Pacific island origin), and genetic factors, including a family history of stroke.

Estimating the risk of a stroke

If someone has any of the risk factors listed in chapter three, then that person is at an increased risk of having a stroke. The more risk factors someone has, the higher the risk. For example, if a person smokes and has hypertension, then their risk of having a stroke is 20 times higher than it is for someone who doesn't smoke or have hypertension. Many people have more than two risk factors.

A simple sum can be used to estimate your personal risk of having a stroke. To calculate your total risk, add up the scores for each of the risk factors present (see chart on page 40).

If the sum is between 1 and 4, you're at a low risk (you have a 5–10 per cent higher chance of having a stroke than a person of similar age without these risk factors, i.e. someone with a sum of 0). If the sum is between 5 and 9, you're at a moderately low risk of having a stroke (a 10–20 per cent higher chance of having a stroke than a person of similar age without these risk factors). If the sum is between 10 and 13, you're at a moderately high risk of having a stroke (a 20–40 per cent higher chance). And if the sum is 14 or greater, you're at very high risk of having a stroke (over 40 per cent higher).

If you set a goal for reducing your personal risk factors and putting their corrected scores in the chart as you go, you'll be able to see your risk of having a stroke reducing.

What can be done about modifiable risk factors?

There are a number of effective ways of reducing your personal risk of having a stroke. The measures depend on your particular habits, lifestyle and medical conditions. Some of them are listed on the following pages.

PERSONAL STROKE RISK

Risk factor	Risk factor score				Current score
	0	**1**	**2**	**3**	
Age (years)	0-44	45-64	65-74	75+	
Smoking	Never smoked or quit more than 5 years ago	Quit smoking less than 5 years ago	Current smoker – less than 20 cigarettes a day	Current smoker – 20 or more cigarettes a day	
Blood pressure (mm Hg)	Normal <120/80	Borderline elevated to mild hyper-tension 120-159/80-94	Moderate hypertension 160-179/95-109	Severe hypertension 180+/110+	
Diabetes	None known	N/A*	Family history of diabetes	Known diabetic	
Family history of stroke	None	A blood relative has had a stroke when older than 65 years	A blood relative has had a stroke when younger than 65 years	Two or more blood relatives have had a stroke	
Cholesterol	Below average (<5.2 mmol/L or <200 mg/dL	Average (5.2-6.1 mmol/L or 200-239 mg/dL)	Moderately elevated (6.2-7.8 mmol/L or 240-300 mg/dL)	Severely elevated (>7.8 mmol /L or >300 mg/dL)	
Alcohol (standard drinks per day)	No excess (0-2 drinks for a male and 0-1 for a female)	Mild excess (3-4 drinks for a male and 2 for a female)	Moderate excess (5-6 drinks for a male and 3-4 for a female)	Severe excess (greater than 6 drinks for a male and greater than 4 for a female)	
BMI (kg/m²)	Normal (18.5-24.9)	Slightly overweight (25-26.9)	Moderately overweight (27-29.9)	Obese (30 or greater)	
Physical activity	Normal (1 hour ener-getic activity at least 3 times/week)	Slightly reduced (1 hour energetic activity 1-2 times/week)	Moderately reduced (less than 1 hour energetic activity once a week)	Very little physical activity (virtually no energetic activity)	

*N/A — not applicable.   **Total score:**
This chart to be used as an indication only.
Modified from The Stroke Foundation of New Zealand Guidelines (2003), with permission.

Smoking

Regardless of how long a person has smoked and the number of cigarettes they smoke each day, the importance of stopping active smoking and reducing any exposure to passive smoking can't be overestimated. It's a common misconception that if a long-term smoker stops abruptly it may adversely affect their health. This isn't true, and the sooner a person stops smoking the more their health will benefit. The risk of a stroke caused by smoking begins to drop immediately a person quits, and after about five years virtually disappears. For health, the best way of quitting is to stop smoking completely — to go 'cold turkey'. However, if you feel that a gradual reduction over several weeks is more likely to work, then do it that way. In situations where it's difficult to stop smoking completely, help from a doctor can make all the difference. Their support can include special nicotine-replacement medications (special chewing gum and skin patches), psychotherapy (including hypnosis) and information about community programmes, including support groups.

Unhealthy diet

An unhealthy diet is a major risk factor for a stroke. These recommendations are a general guideline to healthy eating:

- Limit the amount of fat you eat, especially saturated fat, which is predominantly found in animal products (e.g. meat and dairy products and foods that contain meat products, such as pastry and biscuits)
- Limit the amount of salt. Don't use table salt and eat less processed foods, including processed meats and salted crisps and similar snacks. Your daily salt intake should be less than 6 g (2.3 g of sodium), which is approximately a quarter of a teaspoon of salt. Our bodies need only 0.5 grams of sodium per day

- Eat more vegetables (a minimum of 5 portions per day)
- Eat more fruit, wholegrain breads and cereals
- Eat more fish, especially oily fish such as salmon and tuna — try to eat fish at least twice a week
- Eat low-fat dairy products rather than full-fat ones
- Reduce the number of red-meat portions you eat and avoid eating visible animal fat and chicken skin
- Minimise high-fat and high-sugar junk foods
- Grill, boil, steam, bake or microwave food rather than frying it
- Use unsaturated plant oils (such as olive, canola or sunflower oils) sparingly in cooking to replace animal fats
- Avoid eating too much sugar
- Avoid excessive alcohol
- Drink more water (at least 8 glasses/2 litres a day).

There's no need to restrict the amount of low-fat, low-calorie, well-balanced foods in your diet (see Appendix 3 for details and recipes). Fasting, skipping meals and severe dieting aren't recommended because they can slow the metabolism, cause an imbalance of nutrients and actually increase the appetite.

Note that some types of dietary fats (e.g. unsaturated and polyunsaturated fatty acids, including omega-3 fatty acids) can improve a person's blood cholesterol profile and reduce the risk of atherosclerosis leading to cardiovascular disease and ischaemic strokes. Some vegetable oils (e.g. olive oil) and fish are particularly rich in these 'good' fats and it's sensible to include them in your diet. Remember, however, that vegetable oils are still fats and if you're overweight an overall reduction in total dietary fat is generally advisable.

The use of meat substitutes, such as veggie burgers, veggie hot dogs and meatless bacon, can be a great help to those who want to reduce their red meat intake but have difficulty giving up the taste of meat.

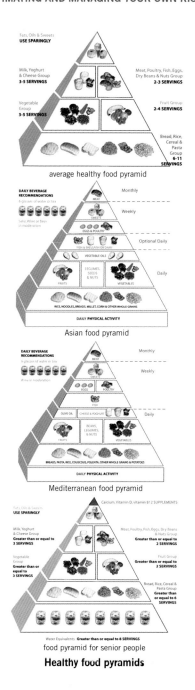

average healthy food pyramid

Asian food pyramid

Mediterranean food pyramid

food pyramid for senior people

Healthy food pyramids

Reducing your salt intake by only 2 g a day can result in a blood-pressure reduction of approximately 4 mm Hg systolic and 2 mm Hg diastolic. There's evidence that salt reduction alone, or combined with weight loss, can reduce the risk of high blood pressure by 20 per cent. To achieve this, reduce the salt you use in cooking and at the table and eat less salty foods, such as pickles, salted snack foods, fast foods, prepackaged convenience foods and processed meats (e.g. sausages, hot dogs, etc.). To maintain the flavour of your meals, replace regular table salt with low-sodium substitutes (e.g. HälsoSalt, Nu-Salt, etc.) and flavour the food with pepper, lemon juice, garlic and other herbs and spices.

It's useful to read the nutritional information on canned and packet foods, noting especially the contents of cholesterol, saturated fats and salt (17 mmol of sodium is equivalent to about 1 g of salt). In New Zealand and Australia, some healthy food products bear the National Heart Foundation logo 'Pick the Tick'. This logo identifies foods low in fat, sugar and salt and high in fibre.

Overall, a healthy diet can decrease blood cholesterol and low-density lipoprotein cholesterol ('bad' cholesterol) and may be just as effective as lipid-lowering drugs, especially when combined with sufficient physical activity.

Hypertension

It's important that anyone diagnosed with hypertension (elevated blood pressure) sees a doctor regularly and follows the recommendations the doctor gives to control their blood pressure. The scope and intensity of these recommendations will depend on the severity and duration of the hypertension and on any other associated conditions.

Modern studies show that the lower a person's blood pressure is, the lower is their risk of having a stroke (either a primary or a recurrent stroke). Each 10 mm Hg reduction in systolic blood pressure or 5 mm Hg reduction in diastolic blood pressure will reduce the risk of a stroke by approximately one third. Even within the normal range, a person with a blood pressure of 114/74 mg Hg has a lower risk of a stroke than a person with blood pressure of 118/78 mm Hg. Most experts recommend people aim to maintain their blood pressure at the lowest possible level that can be well tolerated. This is particularly important for people with diabetes or chronic kidney disease.

At the initial stages of mild hypertension (systolic blood pressure within 120–139 mm Hg and/or diastolic blood pressure within 80–89 mm Hg), altering your lifestyle may be sufficient to control your blood pressure — bring it down to 120/80 mm Hg or below. These changes may include losing weight, altering your diet, increasing your level of exercise and stopping smoking (including reducing your exposure to passive smoking). If following these recommendations for 3 months doesn't bring your blood pressure under control, then your doctor may recommend blood-pressure lowering medications (antihypertensives).

The first line of treatment for people with mild, uncomplicated hypertension is usually thiazide diuretics (drugs that cause fluid loss), with other drugs added as necessary.

Most people with more severe hypertension need two or more drugs to lower their blood pressure. There are five main types of antihypertensive drug:

- diuretics (e.g. bendrofluazide)
- beta-blockers (e.g. atenolol) and alpha-blockers (e.g. labetalol)
- angiotensin-converting enzyme (ACE) inhibitors (e.g. perindopril, captopril, quinapril, enalapril, ramipril)
- angiotensin 2 receptor blockers (e.g. telmisartan, candesartan)
- calcium-channel blockers (e.g. diltiazem, felodipine).

Once blood-pressure medication is started it needs to be continued and monitored without any breaks for the rest of that person's life. Any alterations in antihypertensive drugs in terms of particular type, time and frequency of intake should only be made by a doctor. In rare instances, lifestyle changes can be enough to keep the blood pressure at the target healthy level, and a person may be able to discontinue their drugs. They should, however, have their blood-pressure level measured at least once every 3 months. It's important to talk to your doctor before giving up blood-pressure medications. Suddenly stopping them can cause a rapid increase in blood pressure that can lead to a stroke or myocardial infarction.

Modern antihypertensive drugs have few side effects, so there's minimal danger in taking them regularly for life. However, consult your doctor if you notice any unusual symptoms that may be associated with the medication, such as nausea, headaches, dizziness, fatigue or a cough. If the cause is related to the medication, the doctor may recommend changing the dosage or the timing of intake or trying an alternative drug that doesn't cause the same side effects. It's important to remember that the beneficial effects of blood-pressure lowering treatment are always enhanced by healthy lifestyle changes, and that unhealthy lifestyle factors (smoking, being overweight, drinking too much alcohol, lack of physical exercise, etc.) always diminish the treatment effects.

Atrial fibrillation

If atrial fibrillation (AF) is diagnosed within a few weeks it can often be cured with either medication or electrical cardioversion (defibrillation), which is electrical stimulation of the heart to convert AF into normal regular heartbeats.

Electrical cardioversion can be painful, so patients are given sedative drugs before the procedure. Since it carries a small risk of blood clotting complications, it's usually

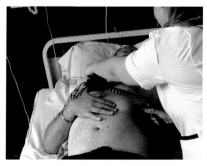

Electrical cardioversion (defibrillation)

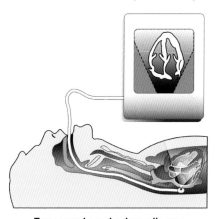

Transoesophageal echocardiogram

preceded by a 3-week treatment with anticoagulants (blood-thinning drugs), unless the presence of a blood clot in the heart can be ruled out using a diagnostic ultrasound procedure called transoesophageal echocardiography. After successful cardioversion patients are advised whether or not they need further antiarrhythmic medication to maintain a stable heart rhythm. Young healthy adults usually don't require long-term treatment. In some difficult cases, surgery with, for example, radiofrequency ablation (ultrasound severing of the communication between the atrial and the ventricular chambers of the heart) followed by the insertion of a pacemaker is recommended.

When cardioversion isn't appropriate or ineffective even after several attempts, AF treatment is usually based on medication that stops the heart beating too rapidly. In these cases, long-term (often lifelong) treatment with warfarin or aspirin is usually advised to prevent stroke-causing blood clots forming within the fibrillating heart. There's evidence that anticoagulation therapy with warfarin reduces the risk of a stroke by almost 70 per cent.

It's important to control the risk factors that can be associated with AF, such as high blood pressure, smoking and excessive alcohol intake, as well as any other stroke risk factors.

Heart defects and heart failure

There are special treatment options for various types of heart failure and heart-valve or wall defects, whether they're present from birth or acquired later in life. These may include medical and surgical treatment (e.g. surgical correction of the affected heart valves or even heart replacement), as well as control of any other risk factors. A doctor will determine the treatment that's most appropriate, taking into account the person's age and other medical conditions.

Atherosclerosis

Atherosclerosis is hardening of the arteries. People with atherosclerosis should take every effort to stop smoking, control their hypertension and avoid excessive alcohol consumption. They should be physically active and eat a healthy diet (see below for details).

Patients who've had an ischaemic stroke or a TIA resulting from substantial narrowing of the carotid artery in the neck (usually by 70 per cent or more) caused by atherosclerosis may be offered a carotid endarterectomy, an operation to remove the narrowing and unblock the artery. Those suitable for surgery are usually advised to wait at least several days or

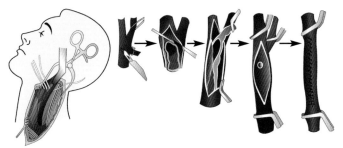

Carotid endarterectomy

weeks after the stroke or TIA before the operation. At present, there's no evidence that the surgery is effective if it takes place later than 3 years after the last stroke or TIA.

After the operation, patients generally stay in hospital for about 2 days. During the next 2 weeks, the patient must refrain as much as possible from turning their head — a stand-up restrictive collar can help with this. The procedure does have a risk of complications, and 5–7 per cent of patients have another stroke or die. A doctor will discuss the risks and benefits with the patient based on their medical condition and the local surgical risks. It's recommended that the combined risk of post-surgical stroke or death should be less than 6 per cent. Women appear to be at a higher risk of post-surgical complications than men. However, this surgery, if done in a specialised centre by experienced surgeons, can be a good option after a TIA or a non-severely disabling ischaemic stroke. Carotid endarterectomy can not only prevent a further stroke (although it's not a guarantee) but can also improve a patient's physical functioning and general quality of life.

High cholesterol

People with high cholesterol are usually put on low-cholesterol diets. If these diets are unsuccessful, medication with lipid-lowering drugs called statins, such as lovastatin

(Mevacor), pravastatin (Pravachol) or simvastatin (Zocor), can help. These drugs help to raise the level of 'good' cholesterol, slow progression or even reverse atherosclerosis and open up the arteries. They're usually taken once or twice a day for many years, and have few side effects. However, these medications are quite expensive and are only effective during the period they're taken. There's good evidence that appropriate lifestyle changes combined with a low-fat diet (especially one low in saturated fat) and a low-cholesterol diet (see Appendix 2) can stop atherosclerosis from progressing even without drug treatment.

Transient ischaemic attack (TIA)

A recent US survey showed that although approximately 2 out of every 100 adults has had a transient ischaemic attack (TIA), only 1 out of 100 of those people could recognise at least one common symptom (see chapter 2) and only 60 per cent of them had sought immediate medical attention. Given the very high risk of having a stroke after a TIA and that it isn't possible to distinguish a TIA from a stroke within the first 24 hours, it's vitally important to get medical help immediately after the development of any warning signs of a stroke or TIA, even if there's only a suspicion of having such symptoms. Identifying and managing the cause of the TIA (e.g. atherosclerosis, emboli from the heart, etc.) can prevent a stroke and cardiovascular complications.

Diabetes

To prevent a stroke, people with diabetes should try to keep their blood-sugar level under control and make sure that all aspects of their health are carefully controlled. As diabetes isn't curable, treatment needs to be continued for life. To keep their blood-sugar level in the normal range and to maintain an appropriate body weight, all diabetics require a healthy and balanced diet with a controlled intake of carbohydrates and fat and an adequate level of physical activity. People with type II diabetes usually need to self-check their blood-sugar levels 2–3 times each week at different times of the day, while people with type I diabetes need to check their blood sugar at least once a day, usually before breakfast and then about 2 hours after a meal. The ideal blood-sugar levels are 3–6 mmol/L before meals and 3–8 mmol/L about 2 hours after meals.

Unruptured intracranial aneurysms

Unruptured intracranial aneurysms are often diagnosed by chance during a brain scan for another reason. However, some people choose to be screened for reassurance. Approximately 10–15 per cent of people diagnosed with unruptured intracranial aneurysms have a family history of them or of subarachnoid haemorrhages.

The existence of an aneurysm doesn't necessarily mean that it will rupture and, in fact, most never do. The management plan depends on a number of factors, including the size of the aneurysm, its location, the age of the person and other associated medical conditions.

MRI angiography is the most common screening method for detecting unruptured intracranial aneurysms or blood-vessel malformations. At present, most stroke experts recommend restricting screening for unruptured intracranial aneurysms to people who have polycystic kidney disease and also a family history of intracranial aneurysms or subarachnoid haemorrhages, particularly those with more than one affected family member.

Screening may be appropriate for people with either a condition associated with intracranial aneurysms or a family history of intracranial aneurysms or subarachnoid haemorrhages, where they have indeterminate symptoms or a high-risk occupation, such as an airline pilot.

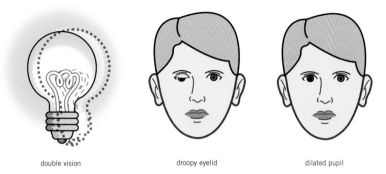

double vision   droopy eyelid   dilated pupil

Some signs of a growing aneurysm

Some unruptured aneurysms leak, grow or both, which can provide help with their early detection and treatment. The most typical sign of leaking is a sudden, unusual severe headache with or without a stiff neck, nausea and vomiting. It's often accompanied by an aversion to light and noise. Signs of an aneurysm growing may include double vision, a droopy eyelid, a change in vision (especially in one eye), a dilated pupil in one eye and seizures. If any of these symptoms develop, call an ambulance as soon as possible.

Being overweight

In most cases, people who are overweight can lose enough weight to be healthy simply by modifying their diet and increasing the amount of physical exercise they do.

If you're overweight, try to eat slowly and take in plenty of water or sugar-free drinks with your meals. One useful strategy is to start eating a third less than usual, and not to eat leftovers. Cutting just 500 kcal (2100 kJ) a day from your diet will result in a loss of 0.45 kg (about 1 lb) a week.

Follow healthy-diet recommendations (see Appendix 2) to ensure you are getting a well-balanced mix of all the important nutrients, especially protein, carbohydrate, fibre and micronutrients. Multivitamin and mineral supplements can help ensure you're taking in enough micronutrients. It's a good idea to get medical advice, especially in the early stages of a weight-control programme. Dietary recommendations are most effective when they're specific for a particular person so, if possible, consult a dietitian or nutritionist who will be able to design the most appropriate and comfortable diet for you.

Your doctor should be able to give advice on the type and level of exercise that would suit you. Choose something you'll enjoy to make it easier to stick with it. In general, your physical activity should be increased to a level that can be maintained regularly. For example, 30 minutes of regular-speed walking burns approximately 40 kcal per 10 kg of body mass, while 30 minutes of jogging burns 55 kcal per 10 kg. This means an 80-kg person taking a regular 30-minute walk will burn 320 kcal, and the same person taking a 30-minute jog will burn 440 kcal.

On average, every kilogram of weight lost can result in a reduction of systolic and diastolic blood pressure of about 1.1–1.6 mm Hg. For example, a weight loss of 5–10 kg in people who are overweight will lead to a reduction of blood pressure of 8–16/5–11 mm Hg.

There are medications that can help with weight loss but they do have some side effects, sometimes quite severe ones, and are only effective if they're used in conjunction with a change in diet and increased exercise. In rare cases of severe obesity (a BMI of 40 or more), surgery to reduce the size of the stomach can also be considered.

Low body weight

Being underweight isn't a risk factor for an ischaemic stroke or an intracerebral haemorrhage. However, if someone is underweight and has other risk factors for a subarachnoid haemorrhage (e.g. they're a smoker, take oral contraceptives or have hypertension or unruptured intracranial aneurysms), they should consider putting on some weight by eating a higher calorie diet that's still made up of healthy foods.

Physical inactivity

Regular, moderate physical activity can halve the risk of a stroke and reduce the risk of early death from all causes by about 70 per cent. All that's needed is 30 minutes of exercise three or four times a week at a level that makes you slightly warm and a little out of breath. It may be brisk walking, jogging, cycling, swimming or gardening. The physical exercise should be pleasant so that you enjoy doing it regularly. This will not only reduce the risk of a stroke but also increase your physical and emotional fitness.

In general, you can increase your exercise level by either altering your daily lifestyle to incorporate the appropriate levels of physical exertion in your overall routine or taking up a regular aerobic or sporting activity. To facilitate the aerobic aspect of the programme (the part associated with improving oxygen consumption by the body), it's important to build up slowly. This will lessen the amount of anaerobic exercise (exercise with a lack of oxygen consumption), which can lead to early fatigue. For example, you could start by walking briskly for 15 minutes twice a day for the first week, then increase it to 20 minutes twice a day for the second week, then 25 minutes in single daily sessions for the third week, 30 minutes in single daily sessions for the fourth week, and finally 40–60 minutes six times weekly from then on. If, during the exercise, you feel unwell, report it to your doctor.

Excess alcohol and recreational drugs

If you think you drink too much alcohol (see chapter 3 for definitions) or have alcohol-related problems, you should cut back or quit drinking altogether. Setting up a goal and cutting back gradually over a realistic period of time (a week or a month) can help. It's advisable not to keep alcohol at home and to avoid unnecessary social situations involving alcohol. For people who require extra help and support, there are a number of readily available services and support groups, including counselling and Alcoholics Anonymous, as well as treatments, including psychotherapy, hypnotherapy and acupuncture. Your doctor may be able to recommend appropriate local organisations and therapists.

Recreational drugs are important stroke risk factors for young adults. It's best to avoid them altogether regardless of whether you think you have a problem with them. As with giving up alcohol, there are many support services available, and your doctor will be able to give you advice.

Sleep apnoea

If you have sleep apnoea (temporary inability to breathe during sleep) or are a heavy snorer, see a doctor for a medical assessment of the problem and to rule out the possibility of a physical cause. Your doctor may be able to refer you to a sleep laboratory for testing. Snoring and sleep apnoea are common in overweight people who sleep on their backs or who have an excessive neck flexion, so losing any extra weight and sleeping on your side with your neck at the correct angle may help. If possible, avoid taking sedatives or sleeping tablets or eating too much food after 7 p.m. Wearing a soft non-restrictive collar at night or using over-the-counter anti-snoring devices

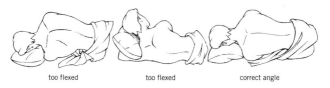

too flexed   too flexed   correct angle

Neck flexion during sleep

and sprays may help, however there's no robust evidence to support the routine use of these remedies. If the problem persists, your doctor may recommend a surgical treatment or the use of a special machine to deliver continuous positive airway pressure (CPAP) through a face mask — this is the only treatment proven to be effective for sleep apnoea.

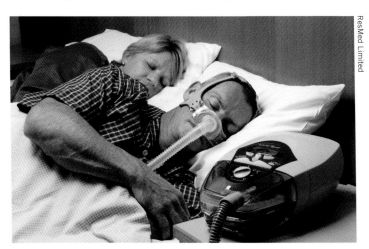

ResMed Limited

CPAP — continuous positive airway pressure

Stress and depression

The best way to deal with stress and reactive depression (depression in response to certain circumstances or events) is to face the problems that cause it and try to do something about them. However, this isn't always possible, and in these situations, it can help to find ways of reducing their effects. The simplest method is to start doing things that make you feel calm, such as walking (especially somewhere you feel at peace), listening to music or spending time with a supportive friend or a pet. Try to think positively and let yourself laugh.

There are also special techniques you can use to control stress, such as breathing exercises, relaxing massage or relaxation exercises, especially those that focus on the face and shoulder muscles. Meditation and yoga can also help. There are many books, brochures and courses available to help you find out more about these techniques, however if you can't control your stress with these methods alone, seek advice from your doctor or another health professional. Anyone with chronic reactive depression or major depression should see a doctor as soon as possible. There are a number of effective treatments, including psychotherapy, antidepressant drugs and cognitive therapy, that can help.

Good sleep patterns are also important in controlling mood disorders. Try to get enough sleep and minimise any daily habits that interfere with your sleep, such as drinking coffee or engaging in stressful activities in the evening, especially if you suffer from insomnia. The relaxation techniques mentioned above may also help. If you're still not sleeping well, see your doctor, a psychotherapist or a psychiatrist as they can help with hypnosis, cognitive-behavioural therapy, biofeedback techniques or by prescribing specific sleep medications.

MUSCLE RELAXATION EXERCISE

To help relieve stress, try doing this muscle relaxation exercise at least twice a day for 10–20 minutes each time. You could, for example, do it before breakfast and before the evening meal.

Sit in a quiet place with your eyes closed, and focus your mind on relaxing each of your main muscles, one by one, starting with the face (forehead, eyelids, cheeks) and slowly moving down to the neck, shoulders, upper arms, forearms, fingers, thighs, calves and toes. During the exercise, try to feel a pleasant warmth in the relaxed muscles and listen to the sound of your breath. When your whole body is relaxed, repeat the word 'relax' silently in your mind at your own pace. With regular practice over a period of time, you may find that you require less time to reach complete relaxation, so the sessions can be shortened and done only when necessary.

Oral contraceptives

Women should avoid taking oral contraceptives, especially combined oral contraceptives, if they smoke or have a history of deep vein thrombosis, heart disease, hypertension or migraine, especially migraines with auras (seeing flickering lights). Talk to your doctor about alternative forms of contraception. If you do take oral contraceptives, you should have your blood pressure checked regularly (e.g. every time the prescription is renewed).

Pregnancy

Women who have unruptured intracranial aneurysms, vascular malformations, heart disease, cardiomyopathy, inflammatory disorders of the arteries, blood disorders or hypertension and who are considering becoming pregnant should consult their doctor before conception. Pre-conceptual counselling, careful preventative care and monitoring are needed because of the increased risk of a stroke.

Hormone replacement therapy (HRT)

Current recommendations regarding hormone replacement therapy (HRT) are that it should only be prescribed for temporary use to treat menopausal symptoms. Perimenopausal and menopausal women taking HRT (especially a combination of estrogen with progestogen) should talk to their doctor about the benefits and risks of HRT based on their individual situation. In most cases, HRT should be stopped if the person has had a stroke, a TIA, carotid artery narrowing (stenosis) or atrial fibrillations unless absolutely necessary. More intensive preventative care is needed if the HRT isn't stopped.

What can be done about non-modifiable risk factors?

Where someone is at increased risk of a stroke because of ageing (they're older than 45), gender (they're male and younger than 65), a family history of stroke or some other genetic predisposition, their modifiable risk factors should be controlled as vigorously as possible. The effect of ageing on the risk of a stroke is greatly diminished if any modifiable risk factors are well controlled.

Specific preventive treatments are available for some inherited disorders associated with an increased risk of a stroke. For these people it's important to seek treatment and to be medically monitored on a regular basis.

KEY INFORMATION

- Strokes can be prevented in up to 85 per cent of people.
- It's possible to estimate your personal risk of having a stroke and to monitor your progress in reducing the risk.
- The most important stroke risk factors can be prevented or controlled. Generally, the best way to lower the risk is to avoid smoking, have a healthy diet and be physically active.
- If you're prescribed drugs that control stroke risk factors, they usually need to be taken for life.

5

The principles
of acute stroke
management

A stroke leads to the death of the affected brain cells, and there isn't anything that can be done to repair the damage once it's happened. However, in some cases, at the very early stages before the brain cells have died, up to 70 per cent of the affected cells have the potential to be saved. There's also strong evidence that appropriate treatment and rehabilitation can significantly improve a person's chances of survival and their recovery after a stroke.

One out of 10 people who have a TIA will have a stroke within a year. Furthermore, multiple TIAs, especially those left untreated, frequently lead to cognitive decline and dementia. Hence it's important to find and treat the cause of a TIA as soon as possible to avoid these complications.

Why is urgent hospitalisation so important?

Modern studies have shown convincingly that early hospitalisation with appropriate treatment and rehabilitation can be lifesaving and substantially improve the outcomes for stroke patients in terms of their level of post-stroke independence and quality of life. There are several reasons for urgent hospitalisation:

■ There are now effective therapies that can save brain cells threatened with death caused by a stroke. These therapies can only be given in the first hours after the onset of the stroke symptoms. Some highly effective treatments, such as thrombolytic drugs that dissolve blood clots and restore the blood circulation to the affected area of the brain, can only be used if the patient is admitted to hospital within the first three hours after the onset of a stroke.

■ Strokes can be caused by either insufficient blood circulation to the brain (e.g. an ischaemic stroke caused by a blood clot) or bleeding into the brain (an intracerebral

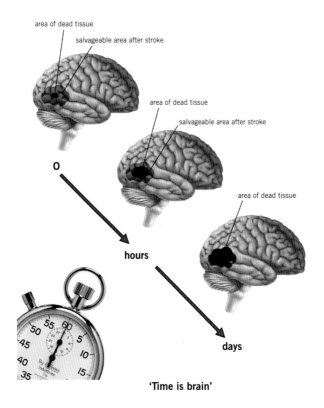

'Time is brain'

haemorrhage) or around the brain (a subarachnoid haemorrhage). Treatment strategies for these stroke subtypes are very different, and the treatment of one subtype (for example, blood thinning drugs for an ischaemic stroke) can be disastrous if used for another stroke subtype (such as an intracerebral haemorrhage). The only reliable way to diagnose stroke subtypes correctly is to use one of the neuroimaging techniques, such as computerised tomography (CT) or magnetic resonance tomography (MRI) as soon as possible. After a stroke, these investigations should be done in a hospital. (Studies show that bedside diagnosis of a stroke subtype based on clinical symptoms alone, even done by a very experienced neurologist, isn't reliable and can result in misdiagnosis in a high proportion of people.)

■ Each of the stroke subtypes can also be caused by different mechanisms, each of which requires a specific treatment. Defining these mechanisms often involves very sophisticated laboratory investigations that can only be undertaken in a hospital. These investigations are also important for patients who've had a TIA because it is necessary to define the cause to provide adequate treatment to prevent a subsequent stroke. Furthermore, some patients who appear to have had a TIA may have actually had a small intracerebral haemorrhage.

■ Quality clinical and laboratory monitoring of a patient's condition is essential for early detection and control of possible complications (e.g. aspiration pneumonia, deep vein thrombosis — see chapter 6 for definitions and details). Specially trained hospital staff in stroke units can provide the best monitoring, prevention and management of these complications. There's evidence that the early management of stroke patients in a hospital stroke unit is associated with a significant improvement in patients' outcomes.

■ A stroke is usually accompanied by other medical conditions that require management by a multi-disciplinary team with the involvement of various medical specialists, such as neurologists, geriatricians, cardiologists, haematologists and specialists in internal medicine (see chapter 7 for definitions and details).

■ The most effective form of treatment after a disabling stroke is rehabilitation. This is best accomplished, at least in the early stages, in a hospital stroke unit. To be effective, it must start as early as possible and be based on a multi-disciplinary team approach, with the involvement of specialists such as stroke doctors, nurses, speech and language therapists, occupational therapists, physiotherapists, geriatricians, dietitians, etc.

What treatments are available?

There are several treatment strategies for people who've had an acute stroke or a TIA. Some of them are stroke subtype specific (e.g. blood thinning drugs for an ischaemic stroke, or aneurysm clipping for an aneurysmal subarachnoid haemorrhage), but some are generic for all stroke subtypes (e.g. blood pressure control and rehabilitation). The members of a multi-disciplinary team of specialists work together to determine the set and sequence of treatment strategies that are most appropriate for each patient. These are discussed with the patient and their family. A GP will be able to monitor the medications once the patient leaves hospital.

What are the treatment options for an ischaemic stroke?

Specific treatments that restore the blood flow in the affected area of the brain after an ischaemic stroke have revolutionised stroke medicine. The treatment may involve dissolving the clot with special thrombolytic drugs (clot-busting drugs), which are injected intravenously or intra-arterially through the femoral artery.

At present, the only thrombolytic treatment with proven effectiveness is intravenous alteplase. However, this treatment is associated with the risk of a potentially fatal haemorrhage, and there are several criteria that must be met before it's used. The most important criterion is that the treatment must begin within three hours of the onset of the stroke symptoms. Treatment given beyond this time is associated with a greater risk of bleeding and the benefits don't outweigh the risks. People who have clotting abnormalities, atrial fibrillation or who've had a bleeding ulcer within the last month are at the highest risk. In addition, this treatment isn't routinely available for ischaemic stroke patients in some countries. A doctor will determine whether it's appropriate on an individual basis and will discuss the associated risks and benefits of the most appropriate treatment with the patient and their family.

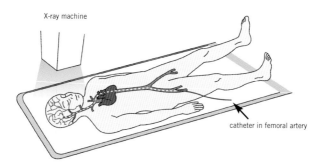

X-ray machine

catheter in femoral artery

Injection of thrombolytic agent

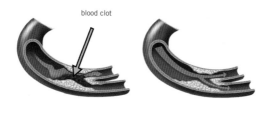

blood clot

Before thrombolysis   **After thrombolysis**

What are the treatment options for an intracerebral haemorrhage?

Most haemorrhages are reabsorbed naturally. However, surgical treatment is an option for some people who've had an intracerebral haemorrhage in the cerebellum and, in some cases, it can be lifesaving. A doctor will explain the surgical

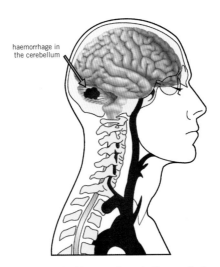

haemorrhage in
the cerebellum

An intracerebral haemorrhage in the cerebellum

procedure and the associated risks and benefits to the patient
and their family, and will advise them on when and where it
can be done.

At present, there's no strong evidence that surgical
removal of non-traumatic intracerebral haematomas in
other parts of the brain can improve a patient's recovery.

What are the treatment options for a subarachnoid haemorrhage?

People who've had an aneurysmal subarachnoid haemorrhage can be given medications (such as nimodipine) to
prevent spasm of the intracranial arteries — a serious complication that occurs in approximately one out of three
patients with this disorder and commonly results in disability
or death. Surgical treatment of ruptured aneurysms is an
effective method of preventing further aneurysm rupture.
People with vascular malformations in the brain may also be
offered surgical treatment.

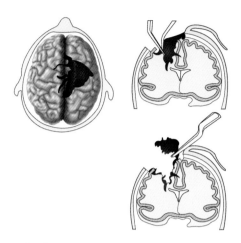

Surgical removal of a vascular malformation

Other treatment strategies

Other treatment strategies for acute stroke patients include:

- maintenance of normal breathing, which may include suction of the airways and administering oxygen
- control of fluid intake and output (maintaining the fluid/electrolyte balance)
- managing high blood pressure
- nursing care (skin care, toileting, nutrition, feeding, etc.)
- elevating the head of the bed, especially for patients who've had an intracerebral haemorrhage or a subarachnoid haemorrhage
- maintenance of normal body temperature (ideally within 36–37°C)
- prevention of possible complications, such as deep vein thrombosis or aspiration pneumonia (inhaling solid or liquid materials into the lung resulting in a chest infection)
- symptomatic treatments, such as painkillers, laxatives or sedatives

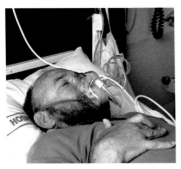
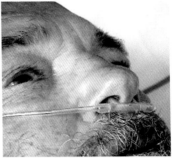

Administering oxygen   Nasal oxygen supply

- the treatment of associated medical conditions, such as heart disease, diabetes or infection
- rehabilitation.

While a patient is in hospital, their relatives may be asked to help with their care. It's important that both the main family caregiver and the patient learn what needs to be done and are actively involved in the rehabilitation process.

Unproven remedies

The promise of a quick improvement or cure sounds wonderful to someone who's had a stroke and also to their family. However, many products advertised this way, whether drugs, herbs or mechanical devices, are expensive and haven't been proven to be effective with regard to strokes. At present, acupuncture, herbal medicine, massage, homeopathy, meditation, soothing music, yoga, herbal medicine, supplements and other alternative treatments should only be considered for controlling some risk factors or as complementary remedies in the recovery phase.

How long is the hospital stay likely to be?

The length of time spent in hospital depends on the severity of the stroke and the number of investigations that need to be done. On average, people who've had a TIA stay in for 1 or 2 days, while people who've had a stroke usually stay in for 2 to 4 weeks. Patients who've had a mild stroke may be able to go home within a few days, while those who had a severe stroke may need to stay in for several months for treatment and rehabilitation. In most hospitals, family members are allowed to stay with the patient during the day and sometimes are allowed to sleep over as well.

What investigations are done in hospital?

Laboratory tests and other investigations are important for an accurate diagnosis of a stroke and its subtype, for identifying its leading cause and associated medical conditions, for determining the best possible treatment and management strategies and for monitoring the progress of treatment. Which tests are actually performed varies from person to person.

CT and MRI

The most important investigations for diagnosing stroke subtypes are computerised tomography (CT or, previously, computerised axial tomography, CAT) and magnetic resonance imaging (MRI) of the head. CT and MRI machines take X-ray or magnetic-resonance images respectively. Each individual

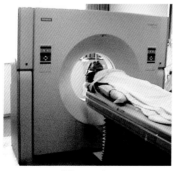 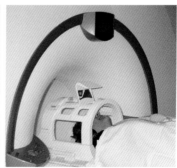

CT scanning   **MRI scanning**

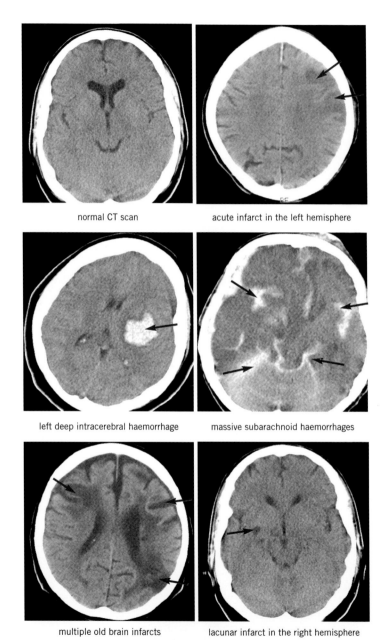

normal CT scan

acute infarct in the left hemisphere

left deep intracerebral haemorrhage

massive subarachnoid haemorrhages

multiple old brain infarcts

lacunar infarct in the right hemisphere

**CT brain scans (right side on scan corresponds to left side
of actual brain, and vice versa)**

image shows a cross-sectional 'slice' of the brain, showing up any abnormal areas within it.

In CT, very low-dose X-rays pass through the patient's head. The X-rays are similar to those used in a chest examination but there's a far lower exposure to radiation. The examination usually takes 15–20 minutes, is painless and carries a minimal radiation risk (except for pregnant women). CT is very reliable for detecting intracranial haemorrhages but isn't very sensitive at detecting minor ischaemic strokes, especially at the very early stages. It can give false negative results (i.e. show no visible damage) for up to half of all ischaemic strokes.

MRI machines use a powerful magnetic field to generate and measure interactions between pulsed magnetic waves and the nuclei in atoms of interest (e.g. hydrogen nuclei) within the head tissues. MRI scanning usually lasts about 30 minutes. It can't be used if there's a pacemaker or other metallic object, such as shrapnel or certain surgical clips, in the body. In addition, some large people don't fit into the MRI machine, while others fear being in a confined place and don't cope with the procedure even after taking sedatives. Like CT scanning, an MRI examination is safe, non-invasive and painless. MRI is more sensitive than CT in detecting minor ischaemic strokes, even at the very early stages, although unfortunately not in every case. It's less sensitive than CT at detecting minor intracranial haemorrhages.

Ultrasound and MRA

Carotid artery scanning is done with ultrasound (using sound waves to create images) or MRA (magnetic resonance angiography, a form of MRI). It's used to look for possible narrowing of the arteries or a clot in the main artery. Both procedures are safe, painless and relatively quick — 20–30 minutes for ultrasound scanning and a bit longer for MRA.

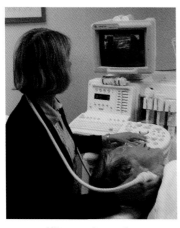

Ultrasound scanning

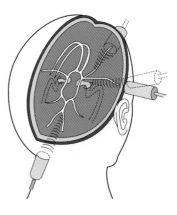

Transcranial ultrasound of brain arteries

MRA is particularly useful for identifying intracranial aneurysms and malformations of blood vessels in the brain.

Cerebral angiography

Cerebral angiography involves injecting a substance that shows up on X-ray images into the arteries of the brain. A subsequent X-ray will then display the blood vessels in the neck and head. The substance used is called a 'contrast agent' (or, incorrectly, a dye), and it's injected either directly into the carotid artery in the neck or through a very long catheter

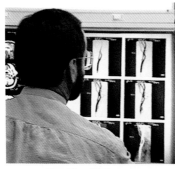

Checking MRA scans

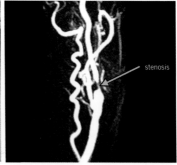

stenosis

An MRA scan

(tube) positioned there via the femoral artery in the groin. Both procedures are done under general anaesthetic.

Cerebral angiography provides the most accurate images of the arteries and veins during all phases of the cerebral blood flow and is used to look for narrowing or other pathological changes, such as aneurysms or vascular malformations. It carries a small risk of complications, however, including another stroke or death in 1 out of every 200 people examined.

Lumbar puncture

Lumbar puncture, or spinal tap, is sometimes used if the diagnosis of a stroke is unclear. It might, for example, be used to rule out an infection of the central nervous system. It's also used occasionally, such as when CT is unavailable, to diagnose a subarachnoid haemorrhage. The procedure takes approximately 10–20 minutes and is done under local anaesthetic. A small sample of cerebrospinal fluid (the fluid that bathes the brain and spinal cord) is taken for laboratory analysis.

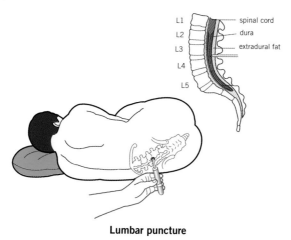

Lumbar puncture

ECG

Electrocardiography is used to look for evidence of an abnormal heart rhythm or heart disease as a potential cause of a patient's stroke. Sensitive electrical sensors, called electrodes, are placed on the skin in particular places. They register the cyclic changes in the body's natural electrical currents that occur with the heartbeat. The results are analysed by a computer and are displayed on a graph called an electrocardiogram (ECG). The procedure usually takes only a few minutes and is safe and painless.

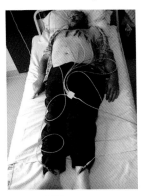

ECG sensors

Echocardiography

Echocardiography is ultrasound of the heart. Sound waves bouncing off the heart are analysed by a computer to form an image. It's used to look for structural damage in the heart, such as valve abnormalities or enlargement of a chamber, or to detect a blood clot that may have caused a stroke. It's a safe and painless examination, which usually takes just 20–30 minutes.

In some cases, a doctor may order transoesophageal echocardiography to determine whether an abnormality inside the heart or the aortic arch is responsible for an ischaemic stroke. This procedure involves placing a special ultrasound probe (tube) into the oesophagus. It can cause some discomfort when swallowing the probe (see page 47), however it's very safe and informative.

Chest X-rays

The chest X-ray is a standard diagnostic procedure used to look for chest abnormalities, including lung and heart disease. For stroke patients, it can also provide a clue to the cause of any deterioration in their condition (e.g. aspiration pneumonia or a pulmonary embolism). The procedure is quick and painless but does require certain precautionary measures to protect the patient from unnecessary exposure to radiation. A lead sheet is used to protect the reproductive organs.

Blood and urine tests

Other laboratory tests used to diagnose a stroke include blood and urine tests. The blood tests may include blood-clotting tests, a full blood count to identify blood disorders and inflammation, an erythrocyte-sedimentation-rate test also used to identify inflammation, and blood-chemistry tests to diagnose diabetes, liver disease, an electrolyte imbalance or other disorders. Urine analyses include chemistry and cell counts to identify infection and kidney disease.

A doctor or nurse should explain to the patient and their family what particular tests are being undertaken and what they're for, as well as the potential risks and inconvenience associated with them. They should also provide the results after the tests have been completed.

All acute stroke patients are monitored regularly, some-times hourly or even more frequently. The medical personnel are looking for changes in the patient's blood pressure, pulse, temperature, level of consciousness (usually by means of the Glasgow Coma Scale that rates the level of alertness) and breathing; they're also checking for urine output, bowel movements and signs of weakness and for difficulties with speech, understanding, swallowing, moving (in bed and around the room) and feeling.

KEY INFORMATION

- ■ A stroke is a medical emergency. It can be treated effectively. Early hospitalisation and quality rehabilitation are key.
- ■ There are general stroke treatments and also treatments specific for particular stroke subtypes. In some cases, drug treatment is accompanied by surgery. A doctor determines the set and sequence of treatments and investigations that are most appropriate for each patient.
- ■ Unproven treatments of alternative medicine should only be considered for controlling some risk factors or as complementary remedies in the recovery phase.

6

Possible outcomes following a stroke

How lethal is a stroke?

Some strokes are fatal while others cause permanent or temporary disability. Approximately 2 out of 10 people who have an acute stroke die within the first month, 3 out of 10 die within a year, 5 out of 10 die within 5 years, and 7 out of 10 die within 10 years.

The more time that passes after a stroke, the less is the risk of dying from it. The highest risk of dying is in the first 3 days — about 12 per cent. The risk of dying within 7 days after a stroke is about 15–17 per cent, within 2 weeks is about 17–20 per cent, and within 1 month is about 20–25 per cent. For those who survive 1 year, the annual mortality is about 10 per cent, which means that 1 out of 10 survivors dies each year.

The risk of death within the first month differs depending on the type of stroke: it's approximately 20 per cent with an ischaemic stroke, 40–70 per cent with an intracerebral haemorrhage and about 40 per cent with a subarachnoid haemorrhage.

Survival after the first ischaemic stroke is about 65 per cent at 1 year, about 50 per cent at 5 years, 30 per cent at 8 years, and about 25 per cent at 10 years.

The long-term prognosis for people who have had a hemispheric intracerebral haemorrhage (a haemorrhage affecting either the left or right hemisphere of the brain) is usually better than with other forms of intracerebral haemorrhages, with an overall mortality rate of about 15–30 per cent. Most people who have brain-stem or thalamic haemorrhages die soon after the stroke.

For people who've had a subarachnoid haemorrhage, the risk of death within the first 2 days is approximately 35 per cent but drops rapidly after that. It's about 30 per cent at 1 week and about 10 per cent at 2 weeks. One of the major causes of mortality after a first subarachnoid haemorrhage is rebleeding. The rebleeding rate is approximately 2 per cent per day during the

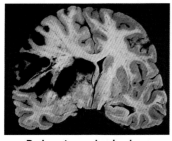

Brain autopsy showing large cerebral infarct

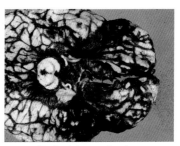

Brain autopsy showing subarachnoid haemorrhage

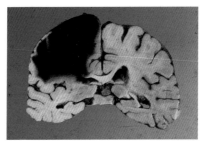

Brain autopsy showing massive intracerebral haemorrhage

first 10 days (giving a total about 20 per cent). The occurrence of rebleeding is a little less than 30 per cent at 30 days and about 1.5 per cent per year after 30 days.

The risk of dying soon after an acute stroke is highest for those who have suffered some loss of consciousness within

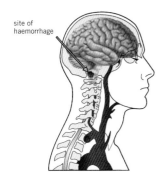

site of haemorrhage

Brain-stem haemorrhage

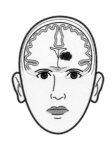

Thalamic haemorrhage

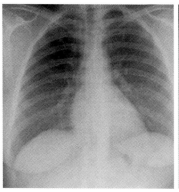 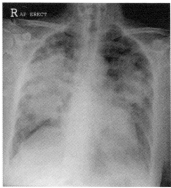

Healthy lung   **Patient with pneumonia**

the first day — the higher the level of unconsciousness the higher the risk of death, reaching as much as 80 per cent in those who are in deep coma, have an irregular breathing pattern or have severe paralysis (complete loss of movement in the affected arms and legs). It's also higher in older people than in young people and in those who are incontinent as a result of the stroke.

Some people who have a seemingly minor stroke die soon afterwards from a second stroke, a heart attack or because their heartbeat or breathing has been stopped by their brain stem, which controls these functions. This is a particular danger in people who've had a brain-stem stroke.

The most common medical complications that can potentially lead to death within the first month after a stroke are:

- brain swelling and subsequent dislocation causing compression of the vital brain centres that control breathing and the heartbeat
- aspiration pneumonia — a chest infection caused by food or liquid getting into the lungs
- blood clots in the arteries of the heart (myocardial infarction) and lungs (pulmonary embolism).

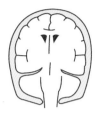

Normal brain
(absence of raised
intracranial pressure)

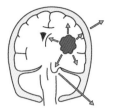

Signs of raised
intracranial pressure
and brain shift

The most common causes of death after 1 year are:

■ infections — urinary tract infections, chest infections such as aspiration pneumonia, and skin infections caused by bedsores
■ cardiovascular complications — heart failure, heart attack and pulmonary embolism
■ dementia.

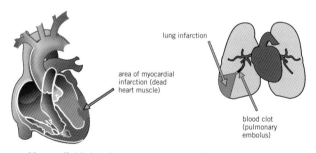

lung infarction

area of myocardial
infarction (dead
heart muscle)

blood clot
(pulmonary
embolus)

Myocardial infarction   **Pulmonary embolism**

Immobilised people with lower-limb paralysis, especially people over 70, have a high risk of deep vein thrombosis (DVT — blood clotting in the major veins of the legs) and a subsequent pulmonary embolism. If no preventive measures are taken, approximately 50 per cent of these stroke patients develop potentially fatal complications.

What are the after-effects of a stroke?

After a stroke, the dead brain cells and any haematomas are gradually reabsorbed. After an ischaemic stroke or an intra-cerebral haemorrhage, they're replaced by a cyst containing cerebrospinal fluid, the fluid that bathes the brain and spinal cord. In most cases, this natural process is completed within 3 months. By that time, one third of the survivors are dependent and may have complications that can result in death or disability.

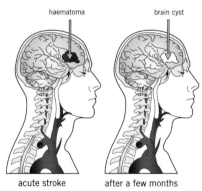

Haematoma reabsorption (brain cyst after stroke)

The after-effects of a stroke include the following complications:

- 80 per cent of stroke patients have partial or complete loss of movement and strength in an arm and/or leg on one side of the body (partial loss is called paresis, complete loss is called paralysis).
- 80–90 per cent suffer from confusion — problems with thinking and remembering.
- 30 per cent have one or more communication problems. They may have an inability to speak or understand spoken language (called aphasia or dysphasia), the symptoms of

which include difficulty thinking of the right words to speak or write, difficulty understanding writing, the use of nonsense words, and problems understanding humour. Or they may have difficulty producing speech, slurring or an inability to make any sounds at all while still understanding spoken language (dysarthria).

- 30 per cent have difficulty swallowing (dysphagia).
- 10 per cent have problems seeing things on one side (hemianopia) and 10 per cent have double vision (diplopia).
- Less than 10 per cent have impaired coordination when sitting, standing or walking (ataxia).
- 30 per cent have problems in right-left orientation and many have no awareness of the problem.
- Up to 70 per cent suffer from mood disorders, including depression.
- 20 per cent develop a pain in the shoulder.
- Less than 10 per cent develop seizures or epilepsy — this is most likely to happen to those who've had an intracerebral haemorrhage.
- Many stroke patients suffer from headaches.
- Without adequate prevention, 20 per cent develop a chest infection within the first month after a stroke, and this is

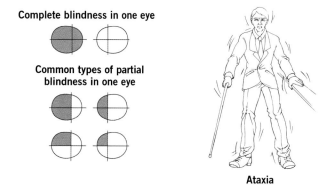

Complete blindness in one eye

Common types of partial blindness in one eye

Ataxia

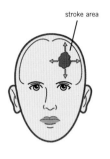
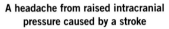

A headache from raised intracranial pressure caused by a stroke

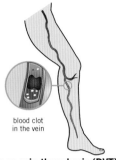

Deep vein thrombosis (DVT)

one of the major causes of death. It's often the result of breathing in food or liquids.

■ Without adequate prevention, 10–20 per cent develop bedsores with or without an associated skin infection within the first month. Bedsores are one of the major causes of death after a stroke.

■ Less than 10 per cent have problems controlling the bladder and/or the bowel, or constipation. This is most likely to happen to people who've had multiple strokes or who have dementia.

■ 5 per cent develop a urinary tract infection in the first month, one of the major causes of death after a stroke.

■ Up to 10 per cent develop deep vein thrombosis (DVT) within the first month.

■ 5 per cent have a pulmonary embolism, where a blood clot breaks away from the leg and blocks a main artery in the lungs, within the first month. This is fatal in about 25 per cent of cases.

■ Less than 1 per cent have a myocardial infarction within the first month. This is where a clot blocks one of the arteries in the heart, causing death of the affected heart muscle. It is, however, more common at later stages, happening to about 30–50 per cent of stroke patients within 3 years after a stroke.

- 30 per cent develop joint deformities and contractures (joints that can't be fully bent or stretched) within the first year after a stroke. This happens most frequently to hemiplegic patients — patients with a complete loss of movement on one side of the body.
- Approximately 40 per cent of people fall within the first year of a stroke, and these people are up to 4 times more likely to sustain a hip fracture than someone who has not had a stroke.

What are the chances of having another stroke?

The chances of having a second stroke depend on the type of initial stroke, the patient's age and their associated medical conditions, especially those that contributed to the risk of having a stroke in the first place.

The highest risk of a recurrent stroke is within the first 6–12 months after a previous stroke. On average, 1 person in 10 has a second stroke within a year, and 3 out of 10 have one within the first 5 years after the initial stroke. However, for some patients with poorly controlled medical conditions (e.g. atrial fibrillation, heart-valve disorders, etc.) this risk is

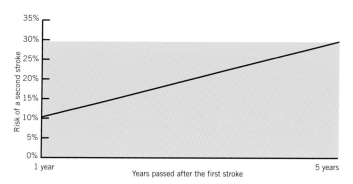

Risk of a second stroke after a first stroke

even higher. The risk of a second stroke can be very much reduced, if not eliminated, if all the conditions that led to the initial stroke are well managed and appropriately controlled (see chapter 4). This is why it's so important to eliminate or control these risk factors as soon as possible after a stroke and to continue to do so.

Many stroke risk factors also contribute to an increased risk of heart disease, which is why some stroke survivors may end up dying from a heart attack if their risk factors aren't well controlled. People who've had a stroke should see their doctor on a regular basis to have their progress monitored. This is the only proven way to reduce the risk of a second stroke.

How to reduce the chances of another stroke

The measures to reduce the chances of having another stroke include:

- Appropriate management of the medical and lifestyle-related risk factors (see chapter 4)
- In some cases, specific medications and/or surgery to treat the cause of the initial stroke.

Possible surgical procedures include the removal of an atherosclerotic plaque from a narrowed carotid artery, clipping of a ruptured intracranial aneurysm, or removal of a vascular malformation from the brain. As with all surgery, these treatments can lead to complications. When appropriate, a doctor will discuss the necessity, timing, and the type of possible complications with the patient and their family.

Patients who've had an acute ischaemic stroke or TIA are often given anti-clotting drugs to prevent a further stroke and other complications related to blood clotting. They may be given antiplatelet drugs, which keep the platelets (the blood cells involved in blood-clot formation) from sticking together.

Such drugs include aspirin, dipyridamole and clopidogrel. In some cases, people are given anticoagulant drugs, which interfere with the production of certain blood components necessary for the formation of blood clots. These drugs include warfarin, heparin and clexane. It's important to understand that none of these drugs have any effect on an established blood clot; they can only prevent other clots from forming.

Treatment with anticoagulants requires careful laboratory control of the patient's blood clotting status to avoid the possibility of a haemorrhage. Someone taking an oral anticoagulant, such as warfarin, usually has a blood test (the INR test) to measure their clotting status once a day or every other day (often in the morning) until their INR level is within the target range defined by their doctor. They are then tested twice a week for the next 2 weeks, and once a week for the rest of the treatment. If their INR level is too high, they may be advised to miss their medication for a day or two.

Treatment with aspirin, clopidogrel or extended-release dipyridamole doesn't usually require special laboratory control, but if you're taking these drugs, bear in mind that they can occasionally cause stomach upsets or bleeding complications. The signs of internal bleeding include easy bruising and black or bloody bowel motions. Consult your doctor immediately if you develop these or any other symptoms. People with a history of alcohol abuse, chronic kidney disease or previous gastrointestinal bleeding are particularly prone to these complications.

Once you start taking antiplatelet or anticoagulant medication, it's important to continue taking it unless a doctor advises you otherwise.

The use of blood pressure lowering drugs in the post-stroke period is extremely important to reduce the chance of a further stroke. There's strong evidence that a combination of blood-pressure lowering therapies (such as an ACE inhibitor with a diuretic) after an ischaemic stroke or an intracerebral haemorrhage reduces the risk of recurrent stroke by approximately one third to one half, irrespective of a patient's age, gender, ethnicity and blood pressure. Treatment usually begins around the time the patient is discharged from hospital or about 2 weeks after the stroke. In most post-stroke cases, blood-pressure treatment must be continued without interruption for the lifetime of the patient.

It's important to remember that both anti-clotting and blood-pressure lowering drugs may be affected by a number of other drugs, including over-the-counter medications — if you are prescribed these drugs consult your doctor before taking any other medication or supplements.

What are the chances of recovery?

Recovery from a stroke is a long process that can continue over several years. Most of the recovery, however, happens within the first 2–3 years, and especially within the first 2–6 months. Therefore, rehabilitation needs to continue in various forms and settings (hospital, rehabilitation service, home, residential care) for at least 2–3 years after a stroke or even longer if a patient continues to improve.

Approximately one third of stroke patients recover their lost functions fully, or almost fully, and get back to their pre-stroke activities and lifestyle within a year. About 50 per cent of stroke survivors younger than 65 are able to return to work. Almost 70 per cent of one-year survivors are independent in their daily-living activities, and about two thirds of stroke patients who survive 20 years after an initial stroke make a full recovery (of the remaining survivors, about one fifth require help with their daily activities and about one tenth remain institutionalised). However, at 1 year after a stroke, approximately one third of the surviving stroke patients still have some level of disability — this is mild or moderate in about 10 per cent of survivors and severe in about 20 per cent.

On average, 6 months after a stroke, 95 per cent of survivors can fully control their bladder and bowels; 90 per cent can groom themselves and use the toilet without help; 70–80 per cent have regained their ability to walk, climb stairs and dress and feed themselves; and 50–60 per cent can safely bath themselves.

The recovery time depends on the type of stroke. Because of differences in the amount of brain tissue damaged, the chance of an immediate functional recovery is usually better for those who've had an intracerebral or subarachnoid haemorrhage than for those who've had an ischaemic stroke. As expected, people who've had a more severe, disabling stroke, such as patients with a complete loss of movement on one side of the body, tend to take longer to recover than less severely ill people. Younger people tend to recover faster than older people, and about 80 per cent of stroke survivors younger than 40 return to some type of job.

People with severe accompanying medical disorders, such as heart failure, renal failure and advanced diabetes, tend to recover more slowly than those without such disorders.

Patients who have had a non-aneurysmal subarachnoid haemorrhage have a relatively good prognosis with a rate of recurrent haemorrhage of only about 2–10 per cent within 15 years.

The prognosis for children and young adults is better than for older people, although strokes are relatively rare in these younger age groups. Speech recovery occurs in nearly all children affected by a stroke before the age of five. Children under two years old with hemiplegia and seizures have a worse prognosis, and most of these children are left with persistent behavioural changes, intellectual deficits, hemiplegia and epilepsy.

People who are incontinent for longer than 2 days after a stroke tend to recover less well. On the other hand, those who are continent at 3 days but can't walk at all after 1 week are very likely to be able to walk in 3 months and be relatively independent in their daily activities.

Other unfavourable signs for recovery include: loss of consciousness within the first day of a stroke's onset; loss of the ability to see one half of space (hemianopia); heart failure; spatial orientation problems; a previous history of stroke; atrial fibrillation; dementia; and severe weakness on the affected side of the body within the first few days or weeks (e.g. an inability to move the shoulders or fingers within the first 3 weeks).

Most of the recovery in the first few days (usually the first 2 weeks) is the result of a reduction in the brain swelling that occurs after a stroke. If there's no recovery in weak limbs within the first 3 weeks, then the prognosis for recovery is likely to be poor. However, there are exceptions to the rule, and every stroke clinician can recall people with amazing and unexpected recoveries long after the onset of their stroke. I remember a 36-year-old woman who had an ischaemic stroke with very severe left-sided weakness that persisted with no improvement for more than 3 months. Intensive rehabilitation was continued over this time. At the beginning of the fourth month, minor signs of increasing muscle tone and movements in the weak side of the body started to appear and continued to improve for the next 2 years. By this time, she was able to walk unassisted and returned to her previous job.

The sooner the signs of recovery appear, the greater the chances of a more complete recovery. Recovery tends to happen quickly in the first days and weeks, but is much slower after a month. People who've had a severe stroke and are not able to sit up for at least an hour, or those who are not aware of their surroundings or able to learn are less likely to have a good recovery from formal rehabilitation. Conversely, people who've had a mild stroke often improve on their own and don't need formal hospital rehabilitation at all.

When active rehabilitation no longer produces any marked improvement it will usually be stopped, but patients should continue to work on their own recovery, which may continue for many years. If the patient achieves a substantial improvement during that period, active rehabilitation may be resumed.

KEY INFORMATION

- Approximately one third of stroke patients recover fully, and this proportion could be greater if adequate emergency and rehabilitation treatment were always received in time.

- The highest risk of a recurrent stroke is within the first 6–12 months of a previous stroke.

- Prevention of a recurrent stroke is effective when done appropriately. Once you start on a medication, it's important to continue taking it unless a doctor advises you otherwise.

- The use of blood-pressure lowering drugs in the post-stroke period is extremely important to reduce the chances of a further stroke.

- The prognosis for survival and recovery after a stroke differs for the different stroke subtypes. The risk of death is highest soon after a stroke, especially within the first month. Recovery from a stroke can continue over several months or years, but is greatest within the first 6 months.

7

Post-stroke care and management

Post-stroke care and management require the concerted efforts of the patient, their family and the medical team looking after them. It's important to note that recovery continues after the patient is discharged from hospital.

When should the rehabilitation start?

Rehabilitation after a stroke should start as soon as the patient's condition permits, as judged by the multi-disciplinary team of specialists looking after them. In some cases it may start within the first 24 hours, in others, it may be after a few days or weeks. Rehabilitation usually starts in hospital, initially in a stroke unit or other ward, then in a specialised rehabilitation ward or centre. It continues after the patient is discharged, usually at a specialised outpatient rehabilitation centre or in the home. There's strong evidence that early management and rehabilitation of stroke patients in a stroke unit is particularly beneficial.

What specialists and methods are involved?

The aim of a rehabilitation programme is to restore independence or reduce dependency as much as possible. However, it's important to realise that recovery after a stroke is often a slow process. On admission to hospital, an acute stroke patient is seen by an admitting doctor, who will determine the initial plan for diagnosis and treatment and will make arrangements for laboratory tests and transfer to a ward. Within the first 24 hours of admission, a patient can expect to be seen by their ward doctor and nurse, and within 2 working days, they're likely to be seen by an occupational therapist, speech therapist, social worker and physiotherapist.

The scope of a stroke rehabilitation programme and the

number of specialists involved depends on the impact of the stroke on the patient and their caregivers. Usually the full team includes doctors (consultants, registrars and a house surgeon), nurses (the attending nurse and the nurse in charge of the unit), a speech and language therapist (if the patient has speech, language or swallowing problems), a dietitian (if the patient needs special nutrition or feeding), a geriatrician (for older patients), a physiotherapist, an occupational therapist and a social worker. All these specialists are also involved in educating the patient and their family or carers.

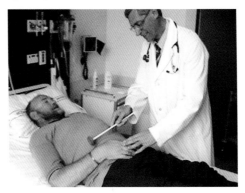

Neurological assessment

A decision is made about the necessity, intensity and location of further rehabilitation by considering the likelihood of improvement, any accompanying diseases, the age of the patient, their family situation and other factors.

A consultant (neurologist, general doctor or geriatrician) is responsible for the clinical assessment, accurate diagnosis and overall management and rehabilitation of a stroke patient, including managing any accompanying medical conditions, such as high blood pressure, diabetes or infection. He or she is usually helped by a registrar and a house surgeon, who provide and coordinate the everyday assessment and management of the patient.

A nurse is responsible for the daily checking and monitoring of a patient's progress, assisting the patient with everyday activities (moving, washing, eating, toileting) and liaising with the treating doctors and other members of the rehabilitation team, including the patient's family. If a patient has urinary incontinence or retention (problems with bladder emptying), the nurse or doctor may use a catheter intermittently or continuously for up to 2 weeks to ensure that the bladder is emptied. If a bladder problem persists, specialist advice from a continence adviser or a urologist may be sought.

A physiotherapist (physical therapist) is usually involved in assessing and treating a patient's movement or sensory disorders, including problems with muscle strength, sitting, standing, mobility in bed, walking, coordination and balance, sensation and fitness. They also carry out physical exercises, assess the range of motion in a patient's joints, and maintain chest and respiratory fitness.

In some cases, physical therapy combined with biofeedback and electrical stimulation (including transcranial magnetic stimulation) can help improve swallowing, gait recovery and arm functioning.

If a patient has problems sitting, getting out of bed, standing or walking, they should remain in bed until the doctor or a physiotherapist has seen them and decided what assistance is required. If a patient needs an aid, such as support splints, a wheelchair, a walking aid or assistance with walking, a physiotherapist can arrange for it.

An occupational therapist (OT) may be involved in assessing a patient's ability to perform everyday activities (e.g. showering, dressing and toileting) both at hospital and at home. This may include assessing the home to ensure it's safe for the patient. In addition, they're involved with teaching the patient and their family members or caregivers the best ways of undertaking daily activities. They also give advice about special equipment that may be of assistance, and can tailor various supportive upper-extremity splints to suit the patient. For patients with severe paresis (muscle weakness), the occupational therapist will cooperate closely with the physiotherapist, nursing staff, speech and language therapist and the patient's family or caregivers to provide retraining in basic self-care activities, such as feeding, dressing and washing. They may also be involved in assessing the memory, perception and thinking processes of a stroke patient and, specifically, their ability to drive a car.

A speech and language therapist should be involved in assessing a patient's ability to swallow food and fluid safely and to communicate with others. If the patient has trouble swallowing, the therapist will give advice on the best consistency for food and fluids and will discuss techniques for safe swallowing. Some patients are recommended for a videofluoroscopy test, which visualises how they swallow some foods and drinks on an X-ray machine.

To prevent choking or a chest infection, a speech therapist may recommend a special diet (e.g. thickened drinks, softer foods), nursing assistance at meal times, feeding through a nasogastric tube (a feeding tube that goes through the nose to the stomach) or percutaneous endoscopic gastroscopy (minor surgery involving the insertion of a tube through the abdominal wall into the stomach). After a stroke, it's best if the patient does not try to eat or drink until their swallowing ability has been assessed and they have been given permission by a doctor, nurse or speech therapist.

People who've had a stroke are vulnerable to malnutrition, which is a significant risk factor for a poor outcome. Other problems apart from swallowing that may lead to malnutrition include a disturbed level of consciousness, motor weakness or paralysis of the usual feeding arm, alterations in a

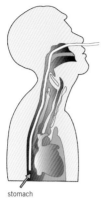

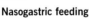

stomach

Nasogastric feeding

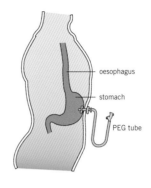

oesophagus

stomach

PEG tube

**Percutaneous endoscopic
gastrostomy (PEG)**

patient's sensory ability and an inability to express hunger or thirst. A dietitian (nutritionist) usually helps a patient by monitoring their nutritional status and arranging for safe and adequate nutrition, including fluid intake. Whereas the speech therapist specifies the diet consistency required, the dietitian advises on the composition of the diet and any specific dietary modifications, such as a diabetic diet, a high-protein diet or additional supplements.

The transition from non-oral feeding to oral feeding progresses through the textures (puréed, minced, soft, standard) and is monitored closely to ensure the patient continues to take in the right amounts of food and fluid. Nutritional support provided by a dietitian to both undernourished patients and patients at risk of malnutrition has been shown to have beneficial effects on post-stroke complications and clinical outcomes.

A psychologist or a psychiatrist may also be involved in caring for the patient if there are any psychiatric or serious psychological problems resulting from the stroke.

Strokes most commonly happen to the older people who have multiple medical conditions, such as heart disease, pulmonary disease and arthritis. The treatment of many such medical conditions is different for older people than for younger people, and so a geriatrician (gerontologist) may be involved in the rehabilitation of an older stroke patient.

A social worker can help a patient deal with the emotional and social consequences of a stroke, including coping with any changes in lifestyle, relationships, work, finance, house-keeping and leisure activities. If a patient needs transfer to other short-term or long-term rehabilitation facilities, a social worker or Needs Assessment Service Coordinator (NASC) will discuss the issue with the patient and their care-givers and help make any necessary arrangements. A social worker will also provide information about local community services and social help agencies.

Where does a stroke patient go after hospital?

A stroke patient's discharge from hospital is usually arranged in consultation with the patient and their caregivers. Where the patient goes next depends on a number of factors, including their current health status, their prognosis for survival and dependency, any associated medical conditions, and their own and their caregivers' personal circumstances and preferences. A stroke patient may be:

- transferred to another hospital or unit that specialises in rehabilitation
- discharged directly home with rehabilitation provided at home, at a hospital outpatient department or at a day hospital. The patient must be able to manage at home safely and the caregivers need to have a detailed knowledge of how to provide appropriate help
- discharged to a residential facility such as a nursing home (private hospital) or a rest home.

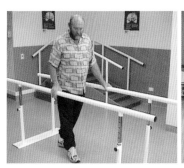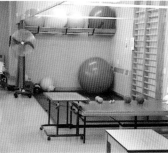

A rehabilitation unit

Many patients who are initially discharged to a rehabilitation facility continue to improve and later return home for further rehabilitation. Wherever a patient goes, they need to be reassessed regularly by their doctor or a geriatrician to see if they would benefit from a further course of rehabilitation in another facility.

Patients have legal rights to full information about their illness and its treatment, to participate in the decision-making process and to make complaints. In some countries, a free advocate service is also available on request. While in hospital, a patient, their family and the hospital staff meet from time to time to discuss any questions related to the diagnosis, prognosis and progress of the illness and to provide other up-to-date information. Before being discharged, a patient and their caregivers will be involved in a discussion with the hospital rehabilitation team about the options and opportunities for the best post-hospital care.

Where necessary, nutritional education is also provided at the hospital. After the acute phase and when the patient's nutritional status is adequate, dietary modifications to address excess weight problems, weight management or cholesterol lowering may be appropriate.

When a patient is discharged, they're provided with a discharge summary, which includes recommendations for further treatment and rehabilitation. The patient's hospital doctor will advise their GP that they're leaving the hospital for home or another institution. If the patient needs further diagnostic evaluation and medical follow-up, their hospital doctor will make appointments. If a patient is discharged directly home and needs some equipment to improve their independence, an occupational therapist will arrange for it. Where they are available, out-reach rehabilitation services are provided for patients who need it so they can continue rehabilitation in their own homes.

KEY INFORMATION

■ Rehabilitation after a stroke should be started as soon as the patient's condition permits, as judged by a doctor, and is better carried out by a team of specialists.

■ Depending on a number of factors, patients who have had a stroke may be discharged from hospital to home, residential care facilities or other institutions, and in time may move on from there.

8

Caring for a stroke patient

This chapter describes strategies and basic techniques for caring for a patient who has had quite a severe stroke.

Before leaving the hospital or other rehabilitation facility, patients and their caregivers need to be aware of all the challenges and responsibilities ahead. Although most patients have made a considerable recovery before they're discharged, some still need help getting out of bed, dressing, feeding and walking. It's important to make sure you know about the local community services that can provide help and support, including your family doctor, a district or visiting nurse, professional or voluntary caregivers, community groups, physiotherapists, social workers, speech therapists and voluntary services. You can keep a simplified diary that includes the patient's medication details and appointment times with the various health-care professionals (see Appendix 5 for a sample layout). It's also a good idea to record the patient's daily or weekly progress (see Appendix 6).

Statistically, the chances are high that a stroke survivor will end up being cared for at home:

- On average, up to 80 per cent of stroke survivors return home within 6 months.
- Approximately 15 per cent of the patients who survive the first weeks after a stroke are eventually transferred to a rehabilitation unit, where the median duration of stay is about 3–4 weeks.
- About half the patients who survive 6 months after a stroke are partially or totally dependent on help with their daily-living activities such as bathing, dressing, feeding and moving about. This includes about 10 per cent of the survivors who need long-term nursing care.
- About one third of the patients who survive for 1 year are unable to regain their independence, and this proportion remains relatively unchanged in survivors after 5 years.

Positioning in bed and physical therapy

The ideal bed for a stroke patient is firm with a headboard rigid enough to take their weight when leaning on it; a single bed enables caregivers to reach the patient from both sides. In some cases the occupational therapist may arrange for a special functional bed for the patient.

It's crucial that immobilised patients are positioned and repositioned properly in bed as this can help prevent complications such as blood-clot formation, bedsores, pneumonia, joint contractures and shoulder pain. In many cases, immobilised patients are looked after in a full-time care facility, however if you're caring for someone at home, it's recommended that you follow these procedures:

- Make sure the patient has a suitable mattress — ask your doctor or occupational therapist for advice if necessary.
- Turn the patient from one side to the other every 2–3 hours throughout the day and night.

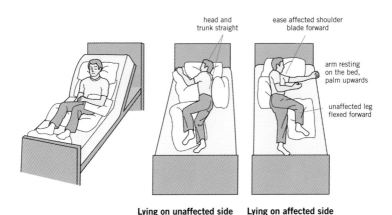

head and trunk straight

ease affected shoulder blade forward

arm resting on the bed, palm upwards

unaffected leg flexed forward

Lying on unaffected side   **Lying on affected side**

Positioning and repositioning for left hemiplegia

- Change the position of their arms and legs every 1–2 hours throughout the day and night.
- Massage the paralysed limbs once or twice a day.
- Move all the joints in the paralysed limbs gently through a full range of slow movements (e.g. straight and bent) 5–7 times. Hold the joint in each of the positions for about 30 seconds. The movements shouldn't be painful. Repeat this process every 4 hours. Where possible, try to encourage the patient to cooperate with the movement, and with increasing their mobility because this will help speed up their recovery.
- Support a hemiplegic (weak) arm with a pillow. Don't lie the patient on their back or pull on their weak arm.

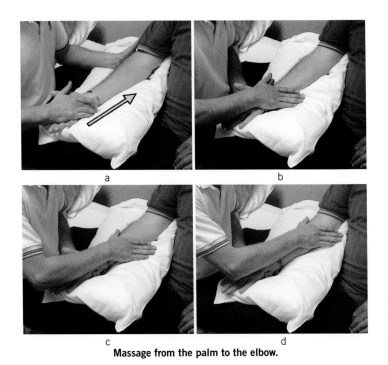

a

b

c

d

Massage from the palm to the elbow.

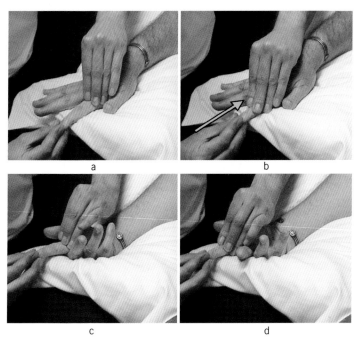

a   b

c   d

Massage each finger from the tip to the base on both sides of the hand.

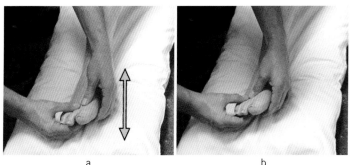

a   b

Massage between each toe where it joins the foot.

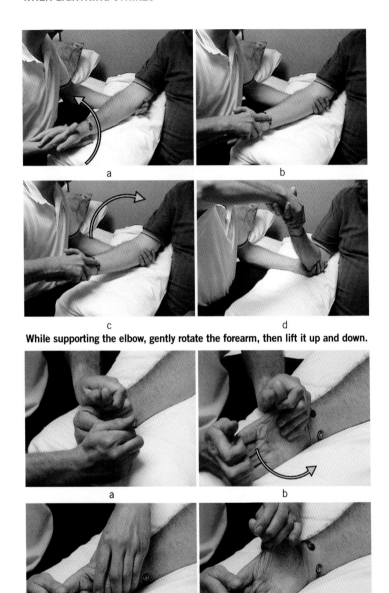

a

b

c

d

While supporting the elbow, gently rotate the forearm, then lift it up and down.

a

b

c

d

Gently and slowly move the joints in the fingers and thumb.

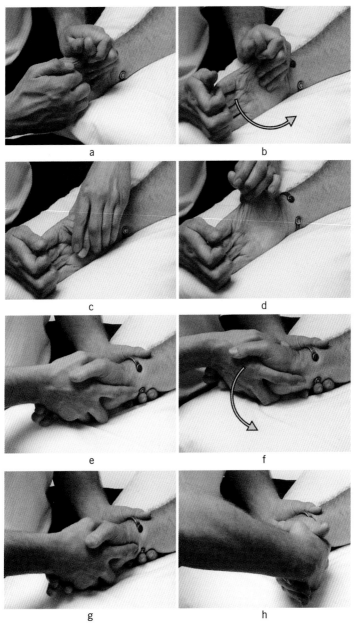

a

b

c

d

e

f

g

h

Carefully move the wrist through its natural movements.

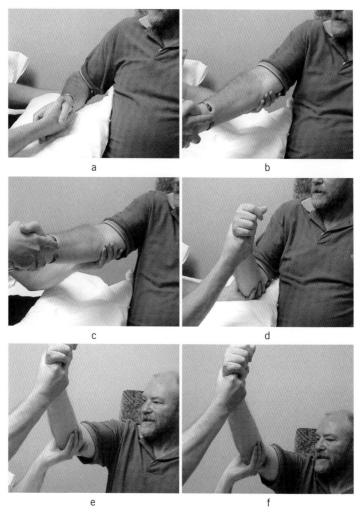

a

b

c

d

e

f

Gently move the arm forward and up in a circular motion.

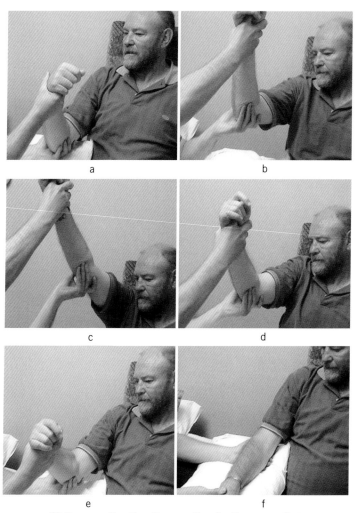

a   b

c   d

e   f

**While supporting the elbow, gently raise the arm so that
the shoulder joint is moved.**

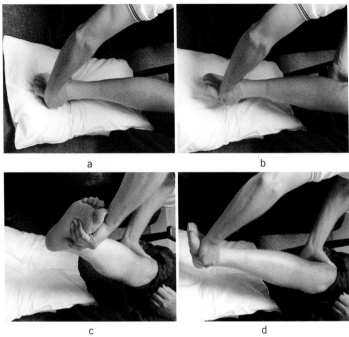

a   b

c   d

While supporting the knee, lift and lower the leg.

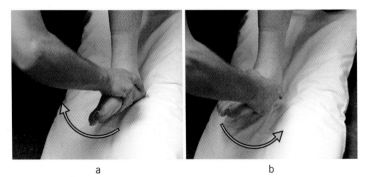

a   b

Gently rotate the foot from the ankle joint.

Turning a patient

It's essential to turn and position an immobilised patient regularly, even during the night. There are some nylon sheets (e.g. Slippery Sam, Slide Sheets) that make moving and rolling a patient easier. To turn the person in bed, the carer should slip their arms under the patient's body and pull them towards themself. Once the person is turned, unfold and tighten the underlying sheet.

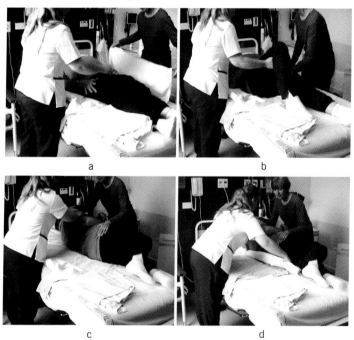

a   b

c   d

Changing sheets around an immobilised patient

It's also important to inspect the patient's back for any signs of bedsores. To help prevent bedsores, clean the skin with warm water, a sponge and some antiseptic or soap at least once a day. Any wet sheets need to be changed straight away.

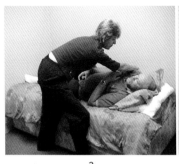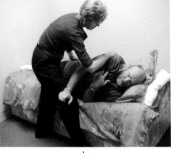

a   b

Moving in bed

Bridging

This exercise can help patients move around the bed. The patient bends up their strong leg, and the carer assists by bending up the weak leg and holding it in position if necessary. The patient then pushes their feet into the bed, and then lifts their hips so that they can then move them to either side and lower them in the new position.

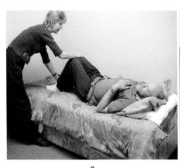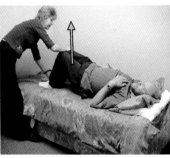

a   b

Bridging

Preventing blood clots

The use of anti-clotting drugs, applying intermittent pneumatic compression, and using graduated compression socks can all help prevent blood clots forming. The patient's doctor should explain if these measures are necessary and provide any information you need.

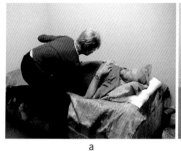 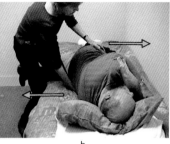

a   b

Turning in bed

Sitting up in bed

Encourage the patient to sit up in bed against the headboard as soon as possible — most stroke survivors are able to do this unaided within a week. They should then spend more time sitting than lying flat. Sitting up is less likely to cause choking and facilitates better breathing and swallowing. If the patient's mobility is severely affected, a hoist can help them move safely in bed. Extra pillows can be used to balance the person and provide support on their paralysed side. At first, one or two people may be needed to get the patient upright, but most people are soon able to do it for themselves. When sitting, pillows should be used to provide support for the weak arm.

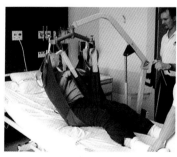 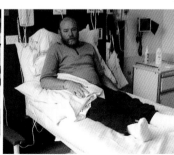

Using a patient hoist   **Pillows support the paralysed arm.**

Skin care

Meticulous skin care is important to prevent bedsores (pressure sores) and skin infections; the presence of these usually indicates less than optimal care of the patient. It's better to prevent them than treat them because they're painful and slow to heal, and if they become infected, they can be life threatening. In stroke patients, bedsores can develop because of decreased sensation and mobility. Incontinence and malnutrition, including dehydration, also increase the risk of developing of bedsores and inhibit the healing process.

Immobile individuals should be turned and repositioned frequently (see pages 103–4), and their sheets should be kept drawn tight. For chair- and bed-bound patients, the parts of the body that are at thc greatest risk include the base of the back (sacrum), the buttocks, hips, heels, elbows, shoulders and shoulder blades (scapulars). Once a day, use a dry sponge to pad these pressure points to prevent the nerves from being compressed and sores forming. While doing this, inspect the skin for abrasions, blisters and any redness that doesn't fade when pressed as these are early indications of bedsores. The patient's skin should be kept dry and powdered.

More frequent repositioning is necessary for patients with contractures or bowel or bladder incontinence, for those who are malnourished or dehydrated and for those who've had bedsores in the past (scar tissue is weaker than healthy tissue). Each time incontinency care is provided, the surrounding skin should also be checked. It's important to clean any areas that are concealed, such as deep skin folds under the scrotum or between the buttocks.

Some bedridden patients may need a special mattress, such as an air mattress. It's important to remember, however, that even with such devices, the carer still needs to turn and reposition the patient and to follow all the other recommendations given here or by a health-care professional.

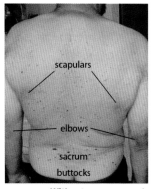

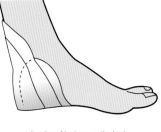

dressing of bedsore on the heel

Without proper care, bedsores can form on pressure points such as the elbows and shoulder blades (scapulars).

If bedsores do develop, their treatment is most effective if started at an early stage. Point out anything that may worry you to the patient's therapist, nurse or doctor. The identification of bedsores by the caregiver is critical for their effective treatment because stroke patients often can't report their presence because of communication problems or because they are unaware of them developing.

Eye and oral care

Anyone who is unable to drink without help should have their mouth swabbed with moist lint or absorbent cotton about once an hour. Regular mouth care is important, especially for patients with poor or absent swallowing.

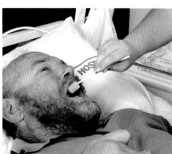

Gently swab all around the mouth.

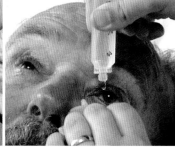

Using artificial tears

Use a clean moist lint to wipe a patient's eyelids whenever necessary. If a drowsy person keeps their eyes open for a long time their eyes can dry out, which can lead to infection and corneal ulceration. To prevent this, eye patching and the use of over-the-counter eye lubricants, ointments or artificial tears (1–2 drops every 3–4 hours) are recommended.

Preventing shoulder pain

Shoulder pain is a common problem among stroke patients, affecting approximately 1 out of 5 survivors 6 months after a stroke. This complication is caused by stretching and inflammation of the weak shoulder joint, and is especially common in people with severe upper- or lower-limb weakness, previous upper-limb impairment, those with diabetes and those living alone at home.

As with many other stroke complications, shoulder pain is far easier to prevent than to treat. In fact, once developed, it tends to persist, often geting worse over time, especially if not properly treated, and it can result in significant disability. The best preventive measures are appropriate positioning and repositioning in bed (see pages 103–4); supporting the weak (paralysed) arm with pillows or armrests whenever possible; avoiding straining the shoulder joint, especially by pulling on the weak arm; and supporting the weak arm with the non-paralysed arm or by wearing a supportive bandage when walking so that it doesn't flop down. Always avoid pulling a stroke patient by their paralysed arm.

Getting out of bed and moving around

As soon as a patient is able, help them to get out of bed and sit in a comfortable chair for short periods of time. The increase in the patient's mobility should be slow and gradual, and, if possible, follow this sequence: moving within bed,

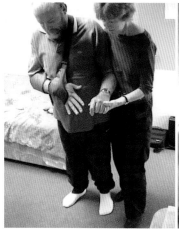 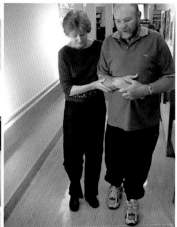

Supporting a weak or paralysed arm   **Supporting while walking**

sitting in bed, sitting in bed with their legs hanging down, standing by the bed, moving to the chair, sitting in the chair, walking on a flat surface.

It is essential for patients to keep trying to get to the next level. Simply lying back and waiting to get better means losing valuable opportunities for the best possible recovery. In this respect, a strong motivation, including trust in the recovery process, is very important. Encourage the patient to try to mentally command their paralysed arm or leg to move and do what they would like it to do. They can use their spare arm or leg to help. The same applies to other lost or impaired functions. As pointed out earlier, nobody knows what makes other parts of the brain take over some of the functions lost after a stroke or other brain injury, but its capacity to do so is huge. For this reason, the patient should never give up trying to recover.

The best indication that a patient is ready to move to the next mobility level is tolerability of the mobility level they're now at; once the patient feels comfortable performing an activity for at least a minute, they can move to the next level.

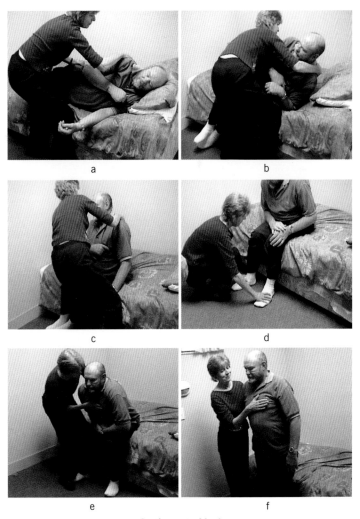

Getting out of bed

For safety reasons, it's advisable to have an assistant or two standing next to the patient and supporting them, especially at the early stages. While standing and walking it's very important that the patient tries to use their paralysed leg by putting their body weight on it as much as they can and by transferring their weight from one side of the body to the

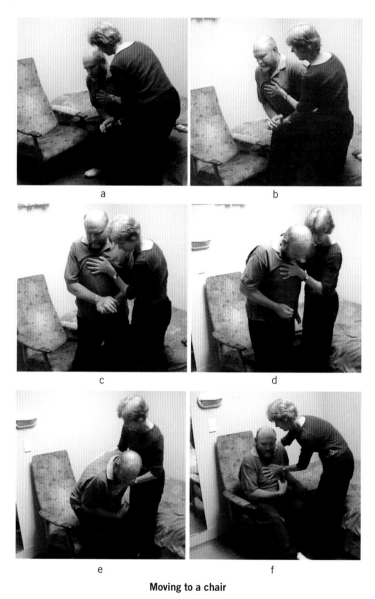

a b

c d

e f

Moving to a chair

other. Patients should attempt only a few small steps at first. Frequent, short practice sessions with slowly increasing levels of movement are the safest and most effective. Once the patient is confident walking on a flat surface, they can start climbing stairs, but make sure the banister is secure and sturdy beforehand.

Even a healthy young person who's been lying in bed for a few days will experience some problems with standing up quickly and walking. People who've had a stroke are often older and their cardiovascular system is often compromised, therefore their tolerance to the increase in mobility can be

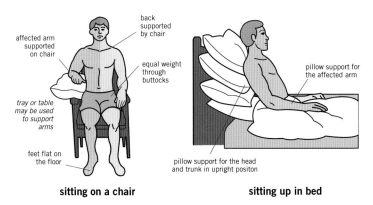

sitting on a chair

sitting up in bed

Positioning for right hemiplegia

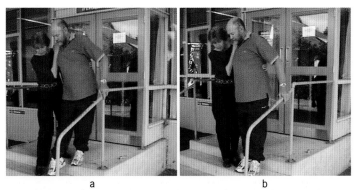

a　　　　　　　　　　　　b
Hold the handrail and, one by one, move both feet onto each step.

seriously impaired. A health professional should advise the patient on whether it's safe to attempt walking and whether they should try to walk alone or with assistance.

Help getting out of bed or moving from the bed to a chair and back may be required, especially at the early stages after a stroke. Place a firm, not-too-low chair near the bed to help with the transfer (if you use a wheelchair, the handbrake must be on to prevent it moving). Remove any small, easily movable rugs or other objects that may cause the patient to slip, stumble or fall.

The following sequence of actions can be used for transferring a paralysed person from a chair to a toilet. Once again, when using a wheelchair, make sure the handbrake is on first.

1. Explain the transfer process to the patient, highlighting the final position.

2. Stand in front of the patient and hold them in a bear-hug grasp with your arms around their back or grasping their lifting belt.

3. Block the patient's weak leg or foot, if necessary, and start counting the lift. This lets the patient know what is happening so that they can give you maximum assistance.

4. Ask the patient to lean forward, then push yourself up and reach for the far arm of the chair.

5. Ask the patient to step around, if possible, or to pivot around so that they're in front of the chair or toilet. They can then sit down.

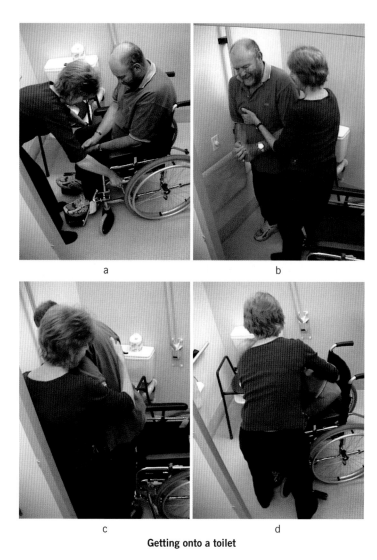

a   b

c   d

Getting onto a toilet

Special care should be taken when transferring the patient to and from a car.

Patients with severe paresis (weakness) tend to slump towards their weak side, but if they stay in this position for a long time, it can cause additional damage to the compressed

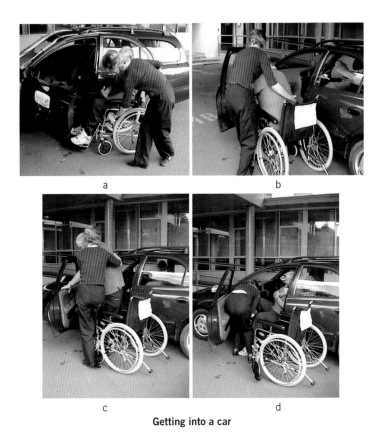

a   b

c   d

Getting into a car

limbs. Such patients need to be checked regularly and their position in the chair corrected if necessary.

Swallowing and eating

Usually a doctor or a nurse experienced at assessing swallowing will observe a patient for signs of difficulty with eating or drinking. The signs may include slurred speech, a wet, gurgly voice or drooping of one side of the mouth. The patient may be given a small amount of water to test their swallowing ability, but this must be done by a health professional. If there are no obvious problems, the patient may be asked to try normal food and drink. If there are any difficulties, a speech therapist can then make a full assessment and determine which consistencies of food and drink the patient can swallow safely.

Swallowing difficulties vary widely from patient to patient. The speech therapist will give advice on the appropriate food and fluid consistencies. You may be advised to avoid certain foods, such as very hard, dry or crumbly items. Fluids can be thickened in a number of ways. Commercial thickeners can be bought at pharmacies and supermarkets (Thicken Up, Karicare Food Thickener, Nesquik NEW Shake, Nestlé Food Thickener, Agar Flakes, Sustagen, instant pudding powder). It's very easy to thicken milk by adding mashed banana, fruit purée or a thick dairy food, such as yogurt. Soups can be thickened by adding skimmed-milk powder, mashed potatoes or other starchy vegetables. Whatever method you use, the food must be smooth and consistent. If you have difficulty thickening food, a speech therapist or a dietitian may be able to help.

If a stroke patient is unable to eat enough food to remain healthy, they may need to be fed temporarily through a nasogastric tube (see page 97), which is inserted through their nose down into the stomach. More severely ill patients or patients who can't tolerate a tube in their nose can be fed via a tube that goes through the abdominal wall into the stomach — percutaneous endoscopic gastroscopy.

Stroke patients need an adequate, appetising and well-balanced diet with enough fibre, fluid (2 litres or more a day) and micronutrients (see Appendix 2 for details). If a patient has a limited appetite, it may help to provide small, high-calorie, tasty snacks every 2–3 hours, along with nutritional supplement drinks (e.g. Ensure, Vitaplan, Complan). To prevent choking and aspiration pneumonia all meals should be eaten sitting up, not lying down.

To prevent spills, lay the plate on a non-slip mat, and, at

least initially, it may help to use a plate with a rim so that the food isn't easily knocked off. There are aids available for one-handed feeding and there are also eggcups that can be attached to a table. Occupational therapists usually assess the need for these and other similar devices.

Managing speech and writing problems

About half of all acute stroke patients have some initial language problems, including slurred speech, but only about one third of stroke survivors continue to have these problems at later stages. Persistent speech problems occur most commonly in patients with weakness on their right side (or occasionally on the left side for left-handed people). These patients may not understand the speech of others or be able to clearly express themselves verbally, or both. Other forms of speech problem include: an inability to find the correct word; the use of nonsense words or, in rare instances, foul words; an inability to speak despite being physically able; an inability to understand written words; and an inability to write.

People with speech and writing problems can easily become depressed or frustrated by their difficulty. Because of this it's extremely important to encourage patients to communicate — accept all forms of communication (writing, signs, gestures, drawings, attempts at speech) rather than demanding clear speech. Use any sign of even minor improvement for further encouragement. Avoid frequent criticism and don't insist that each word be produced perfectly. Instead, try to give the patient a reasonable amount of time to respond to your questions and downplay any errors.

For people with impaired speech and writing, a speech therapist can set up a specific treatment programme for speech and language. Caregivers may be asked to help by providing opportunities for the patient to listen to others speaking or to try to communicate by writing, drawing, giving yes/no responses, making gestures or using eye contact and facial expressions. It can help to talk about family issues with the patient, show and discuss photographs of familiar places or people, chat about friends, or to work through exercises involving repeating words. It's often helpful to figure out the best ways of communicating everyday needs quickly. A speech therapist can give advice on any supportive aids that may help.

Encourage the patient to be as independent as possible and to take part in normal activities, such as dinner with the family or guests. Try not to ignore them during group conversations — they should be involved in family decision-making as much as possible and be kept informed of events. At the same time, try not to burden them with day-to-day problems that will leave them tired or stressed.

People who have difficulty finding the right words should feel free to use other methods to get their meaning across. Instead of saying the word 'library', for example, they could say 'the place where you borrow books'; if the word is 'piano', they could demonstrate playing the piano; if the word is 'apple', they could say 'a type of fruit'. Other methods of getting the meaning across include spelling the word or part of it, writing the word, drawing a picture of it, or pointing to it if it's a nearby object. Some patients find it useful to point at pictures displayed on a board or to write using a keyboard. It can also be extremely helpful if the patient visualises the thing they're trying to name (i.e. forms a mental picture of it).

Stroke patients who can read, write and understand the speech of others but have difficulty saying words clearly themselves (patients with dysarthria) can benefit from doing the following lip and tongue exercises twice a day.

Lip and tongue exercises

Repeat each action 10 times during a session.

- Round your lips
- Smile
- Alternate rounding the lips and smiling, as if you're saying 'oo — ee'
- Open your mouth wide, then purse the lips as if you're kissing
- Throw a kiss
- Close the lips tightly as if you're saying 'mm'
- Say 'ma ma ma ma' as fast as possible
- Say 'me me me me' as fast as possible
- Close your lips tightly and puff up your cheeks with air; hold the air inside your cheeks for 5 seconds, then release it
- Try to touch your chin with the tip of your tongue
- Try to touch your nose with the tip of your tongue
- Extend your tongue out as far as possible, hold it for 3 seconds, then pull it back into your mouth
- Touch the corners of your mouth with your tongue, moving your tongue quickly from right to left, and back again
- Circle your lips with your tongue
- Say the sound 'ta-ta-ta' with increasing speed
- Press your tongue against your upper gums, then against your lower gums
- 'Brush' your teeth with your tongue
- Point your tongue into your right cheek and then your left, pressing it as hard as you can.

While talking to the patient, sit facing them directly, try to talk slowly and use short, simple sentences. Supportive gestures and facial expressions can be helpful. Repeat yourself if necessary and avoid showing impatience or irritation. Turn off any distracting external noises such as radios, stereos or televisions. It's also easier for the patient if other people in

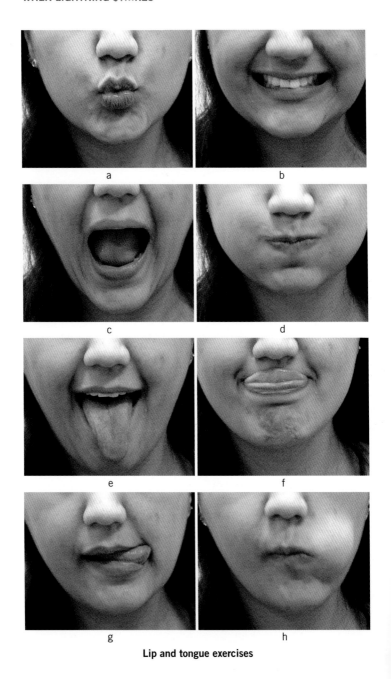

Lip and tongue exercises

the room avoid talking at the same time. Don't pretend to understand the patient when it's not the case, and never insult the patient by speaking about them as if they were not present.

These sessions should take place as often as possible but shouldn't go on for too long because patients with language problems tire easily. A speech therapist can sometimes refer people with communication problems for special individual or group sessions, and sometimes a person who's had a stroke may be matched with a volunteer or be able to join a communication group.

Bladder and bowel control

Although bladder and bowel problems (incontinence or retention) are relatively common in the first few weeks after a stroke, especially in confused or drowsy people, most people recover full control within a few weeks.

When repositioning a patient, it's important to change wet or soiled incontinence pads. Some men can be kept dry by using a urine bottle regularly. Place the penis in the spout whenever necessary. In some cases, however, a catheter (tube) may be inserted in the bladder, and it will automatically drain away the urine. Some incontinent women can be kept dry with the use of incontinence pads, but if this isn't possible or effective enough, a catheter may be inserted into the bladder. Caregivers can be taught how to clean a catheter, but a nurse should help insert it.

Intermittent use of catheters is an option for people with persistent urinary incontinence or retention, however if a catheter is used for a week or longer there's an increased risk of contracting a urinary tract infection, which can sometimes lead to serious complications such as potentially fatal sepsis (blood poisoning). Because of this, frequent temporary catheterisation accompanied by occasional antiseptic bladder

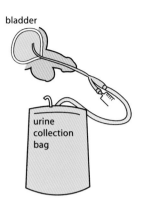

bladder

urine collection bag

A catheter

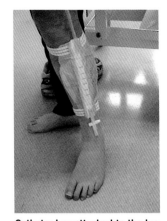

Catheter bag attached to the leg

irrigation is often recommended. If a urinary tract infection does develop, a doctor will usually prescribe an antibiotic treatment to clear it up.

As with anyone else, it's important that stroke patients have regular bowel movements with at least one bowel-emptying every 2–3 days. Constipation is commonly defined as an infrequent passing of stools (less than 3 times weekly) or difficulty with bowel movements. It's a common problem among older people and in people who've had a stroke. Some medications (e.g. opioids) can also cause constipation. The consequences of constipation include discomfort, diminished quality of life and, in severe cases, poor health, including bowel perforation and cardiovascular complications, leading to hospitalisation. The best way to regulate bowel movements is an adequate, well-balanced diet with plenty of fluids (at least 2 litres a day) and fibre (fruits and vegetables) and also sufficient physical activity. Stool softeners (laxatives), suppositories and enemas can be used for occasional constipation, however if the problem persists the patient or their carer should seek advice from a doctor or community continence nurse.

Breathing exercises

For bedridden stroke patients and those with severely restricted mobility, it's important to maintain adequate ventilation of the lungs to prevent a chest infection. This can be done by a combination of deep breathing exercises, proper positioning (see pages 103–4) and spitting out any excess mucus from the mouth. If a patient has breathing problems, chest physiotherapy can also keep the lungs clear.

Managing sensory problems

A stroke can affect the senses in a number of ways. Losing sensation in one part of the body, such as an arm or leg, does not usually affect the patient's daily routine, but they must be careful not to cut themselves while shaving or cooking or to burn themselves with hot bath water or hot objects.

Patients who lose half their vision (hemianopia) or have spatial orientation problems can suffer frustrating difficulties because they're often unaware of things on their affected side. They may, for example, dress or undress only one side of their body, eat the food on only one half of the plate or write on only one side of a page. These patients don't usually learn to move their head to look to the affected side, and so are at risk of getting lost and disoriented. They tend to walk into objects on their affected side and don't see, or recognise, moving objects such as cars coming from that direction. As well as being unable to drive a car, these people may need assistance with walking along the street and many other everyday activities. Sometimes these symptoms are the only consequences of stroke but these patients are still considered severely disabled.

Patients with spatial orientation problems may also neglect noises coming from the left, ignore or deny their left side, even if it's severely paralysed, or may not be able to recognise

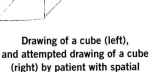

Drawing of a clock by a patient with spatial orientation problems

Drawing of a cube (left), and attempted drawing of a cube (right) by patient with spatial orientation problems

the face of a close relative or spouse. For some patients, even those without paralysis, performing the complex consecutive movements needed to carry out a particular task, such as dressing or making a cup of coffee, is very difficult or impossible. Family members need to be aware of these problems and appreciate that they're the consequences of the stroke and not whims of the patient.

There are things you can do to help manage these problems. For example, a full-length mirror will help the patient see both sides of their body. Touching the affected side to remind them about it may help reinforce the rehabilitation. When talking to the person, it's advisable to stand in front of them or on their good side. Place their food plate towards the good side as well.

A small proportion of stroke patients develop 'central' pain, which is caused by damage to an area in the mid-brain called the thalamus, a deep region of the brain that acts as a sensory relay centre. This pain is a mixture of sensations, including heat and cold, and is often described as burning, shooting or sharp stabbing feelings in a paralysed part of the body. It's often worst in the hands and feet, and can sometimes be very severe. It can be brought on or worsened by even light rubbing of the affected part of the body, by movement and by temperature changes, especially cold temperatures. This serious complication of a stroke is difficult to manage, and consultation with a neurologist should be sought.

Managing daily living

After a stroke, it's important for the patient to resume their previous activities as much as possible. They need to try to get out and start doing the things they enjoyed before the stroke as soon as their doctor permits. It's extremely important to remain positive about the recovery. If a full recovery isn't possible, then at least a partial recovery is almost certainly achievable.

Take care to ensure that the patient's usual daily activities can still be performed safely and make any necessary adjustments. At first, it can be a good idea to practise some activities with guidance from a therapist or nurse. This might include such things as dressing, taking a shower, cooking or using the stairs. When caring for someone who has had a stroke, be careful not to compromise their self-respect. Encourage them to do things for themselves if they are able to.

Patients with spatial orientation problems or apraxia often need help dressing because they're unable to use both arms properly, even if they don't have any obvious weakness in their limbs. They sometimes put their clothes on in the wrong place and often can't manage buttons. When helping someone dress, take care not to stretch any paralysed joints, especially the shoulder joint. Encourage the patient to dress themself as much as possible. It may help to adapt the patient's clothing — buy shoes without laces, Velcro fastening shirts, etc. — but make sure the patient is comfortable with these adaptations before going ahead. Remember that false teeth shouldn't be left in at night, and that they should be cleaned before being put in.

If muscle spasticity is a problem after a stroke, it can be reduced by heating or cooling or by passive and active stretching exercises that work through the range of motions usually performed by the affected muscle and joint. However, if you suspect the patient cannot feel a particular movement,

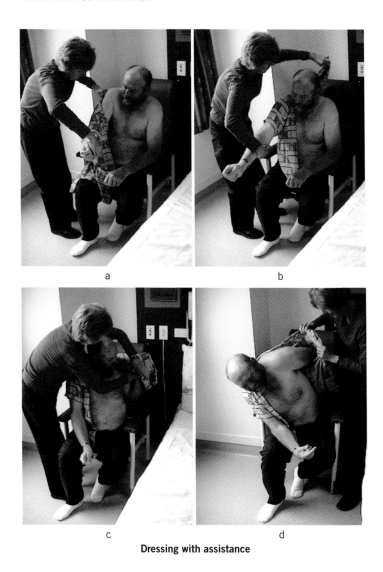

a   b

c   d

Dressing with assistance

take extra care not to over-stretch or damage the joint. The patient's physiotherapist should be able to give you advice on how to do these exercises safely. If these measures are not effective enough, the physiotherapist may prescribe electrical stimulation of the muscles, muscle relaxants (e.g. baclofen, botulinum toxin injections) or other interventions.

If a patient is unable to safely undertake some daily activities on their own, there are special aids and services that can help, including adaptations that can be made to the patient's home. These are recommended by an occupational therapist, who can help make the necessary arrangements. Helpers from social and community services can organise some personal care, including looking after the home, making the patient's bed, arranging 'meals-on-wheels', shopping and collecting prescriptions.

When a stroke patient goes out for the first few times, it's often a good idea if someone else accompanies them, at least until they're confident they can manage safely on their own.

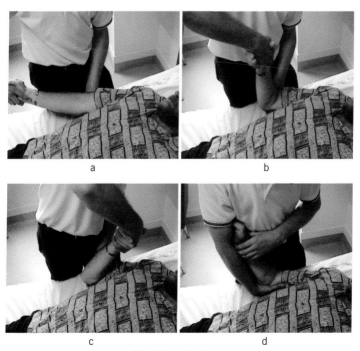

a   b

c   d

Exercising the elbow

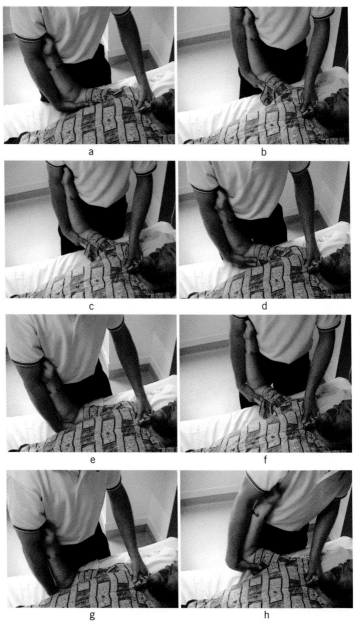

Exercising the shoulder

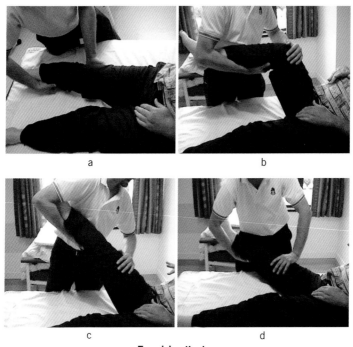

Exercising the leg

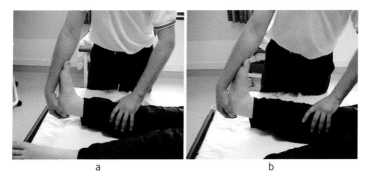

Exercising the foot

If 4–6 months after a stroke a patient can't walk unaided or feels uncomfortable doing so, a walking frame or other walking aid such as a manual or electric wheelchair may be able to provide them with some independence. There are also

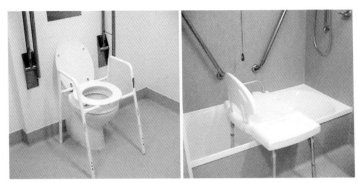

Some possible bathroom adaptations

adaptations that can be made to the patient's car — there are even cars available that have been specially adapted for people with different disabilities. Before actually getting one of these aids, however, it's a good idea to get an opinion from a physiotherapist or occupational therapist about the level of mobility the patient is most likely to achieve and, therefore, find out what aids would suit them best.

If the patient is using a wheelchair and their home has stairs, it may help to install a concrete entrance ramp or a wooden ramp. You may also need to widen household doorways to allow the person to move freely about the house. Installing secure electrical cords, bathroom handrails and other home adaptations can also help.

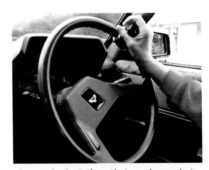

One of several adaptations that can be made to a car

Physical activity, specifically exercises that increase lower-leg strength and balance, may help prevent falls. These types of exercises need to be taught and supervised by a physiotherapist or a specially trained nurse. Some patients experience fatigue during the day, and regular time out or rest periods may alleviate the problem.

Physical activity after a stroke

Safe and enjoyable exercise after a stroke is important for general health and to reduce the risk of further strokes. It's important to consider the level of exercise that was taken before the stroke when planning an exercise regimen. It's generally safest to start slowly and gradually increase the amount and intensity of exercise. The types of activity that will be possible depend on the effects of the stroke. Those with few physical problems can consider walking, using a cycling machine and their usual sporting activities. More severely affected patients, such as those with hemiplegia, may need help from a physiotherapist or exercise specialist. In general, as for everybody, it's best to do about half an hour of activity that leaves you feeling comfortably warm, slightly puffed and a bit sweaty, three times a week or more. Usually aerobic exercise, such as walking or cycling, is particularly beneficial, however the use of weights and repetitive muscle strengthening activities can also be helpful.

Stroke patients who also have heart problems need to make sure their heart condition is stable before changing their usual level of activity. In this situation, it's best to get a checkup from your doctor and discuss your planned activity levels.

Managing emotional problems

Up to 70 per cent of stroke survivors suffer from some form of emotional problem, such as a grief reaction, irritability, unhappiness, sadness or depression. There's evidence that people suffering from post-stroke depression are three times more likely to die within 10 years than stroke patients without depression — this includes death from suicide. However, if the patient and their carers are aware of the problem there are usually things that can be done to alleviate it.

Some emotional problems develop immediately after a stroke because of actual damage to the brain. For example, a person's inability to express themselves because of language problems can lead to irritability. Other emotional problems develop at some later stage, such as when the person finally realises the full impact of the stroke on their independence.

It's important to remember that people who've had a stroke are particularly vulnerable to changes in their situation, especially when they're about to leave hospital or when they first leave home for an outing. It's a normal physiological reaction, and the patient should be encouraged to discuss their concerns with their carers and family members so that the problems can be rectified as much as possible.

In most cases, emotional problems diminish over time, but while present they can lead to a refusal of treatment or a lack of motivation for the rehabilitation process, which can affect the patient's recovery. These reactive emotional problems can often be helped substantially by encouraging the patient to talk about their fears and anger. A patient must feel that they're a valuable member of the family. The importance of a supportive home environment that encourages interest in other people and leisure activities, such as reading, cooking, walking, shopping, playing games and talking, can't be overestimated. Stroke patients whose family or caregivers aren't supportive and who have a dysfunctional home life tend to do worse than other patients. Some stroke patients may be comforted by sharing their experience with other stroke survivors (a list of stroke support groups can be obtained from your local community service organisation).

If necessary, emotional problems can be treated with individual counselling or group therapy. Psychotherapy may also help some people, such as those with severe apathy, depression, indifference or opposition to treatment. If the problems persist, especially depression, a doctor may recommend antidepressant drugs (e.g. fluoxetine and amitriptyline) or consulting a psychiatrist or a clinical psychologist. An early consultation is usually recommended for severely depressed people, especially those who may be considering suicide.

Some stroke survivors, especially older people who've had multiple strokes, have uncontrollable outbursts of emotion, such as laughing, crying or displays of irritation, for no obvious reason. It's important for recovering people and their families to realise that most behavioural problems that develop as a direct result of stroke don't last very long and that they often don't express the person's true feelings.

Managing cognitive problems

Cognitive problems include difficulty thinking, concentrating, remembering, making decisions, reasoning, planning and learning. These are common stroke complications, affecting approximately 64 per cent of all survivors and leading to dementia in 1 out of 5 older stroke survivors. For many stroke patients, however, mild cognitive problems tend to settle down over time and their abilities recover fully.

If a patient has memory problems and is taking a number of long-term medications, it can be useful to have the pills pre-packed at the pharmacy. There are several commercially available packages, such as Blister Pak, Webster Pak or Medico Pac, in which the pills are divided up and labelled clearly so the patient can see whether or not they've taken that day's quota. If a patient can't follow the instructions on their prescribed medications, a caregiver needs to ensure that the right amounts are being taken at the right times. There's evidence that reminders can improve a patient's ability to take their medication regularly. It can help to chart the patient's daily activities, medications and progress on a worksheet, chart or table (see Appendices 5 and 6).

Stroke patients with severe cognitive problems, such as dementia, rarely recover fully and can get worse over time. This is especially likely with older people who've had several strokes and also have other medical conditions.

Some stroke patients are not aware of their cognitive problems, which makes them vulnerable to accidents and becoming lost. Family members and caregivers need to be aware of this and take some precautions, such as hiding potentially harmful objects and accompanying the patient on outings. A consultation with a clinical psychologist or psychiatrist can also help. If the safety of the patient at home becomes a real concern, consideration should be given to transferring the patient to a residential care facility.

Although there's still no effective specific treatment for vascular dementia, it may be possible to influence the development or progression of the disease by controlling the stroke risk factors, particularly hypertension and sources of emboli.

Preventing falls

The risk factors for patients falling include problems with gait and balance, sedative medications, difficulty performing everyday activities, inactivity, incontinence, visual impairment and reduced lower-limb strength.

There are several non-pharmacological ways to reduce the risk of a fall.

■ Older people and those who experience dizziness, a sensation of light-headedness, unsteadiness or visual problems when moving their head or body (especially when getting out of bed and standing) should be careful when moving and avoid rapidly changing their body or head position. Get out of bed slowly and in steps: first move so you're lying on your side near the edge of the bed, then sit up, next swing your legs around so they touch the floor, then stand up, and finally start walking. Avoid rapid head movements, for example when shaving or combing your hair, and avoid bending your head to extreme positions.

- Many older people's falls are caused by dehydration so an adequate fluid intake is very important. Usually 2 litres a day is enough, unless a doctor advises otherwise.

- Physical activity, specifically exercises that increase lower-leg strength and balance, may help prevent falls. These types of exercises need to be taught and supervised by a physiotherapist or specially trained nurse.

It's a good idea for at-risk patients to be taught how to fall safely by a physiotherapist, in case the precautions fail. To further reduce the risk of a fall, some people need assistance getting out of bed or moving from the bed to a chair.

People at a high risk of falling and who live alone can summon help if they have a 24-hour personal alarm linked to a professional monitoring station (e.g. MASS Healthcare, Chubb Medical) or directly with the ambulance service (e.g. St John Lifelink Medical Alarm). These units can be worn wristwatch style, as a necklace or be clipped to clothing, and are activated by pushing a button. They contain a powerful loudspeaker and a sensitive microphone so that hands-free two-way communication is established when calls are made. Some devices have a built-in fall detector that automatically triggers a call for help if the wearer's movements indicate that they may have fallen.

9

Commonly asked questions

What is the family's role?

When it comes to caring for a stroke patient, their 'family members' can include their extended family, or whanau, caregivers and close friends. The family's role in the patient's post-stroke rehabilitation is enormous but the family members should receive psychosocial and practical support at every stage. Hospital staff should be able to supply straightforward information on how to care for and support the patient and will also be able to set up a partnership for solving problems.

It can be a huge help if the family member closest to the patient observes how the health personnel assist the patient and practises under the supervision of a nurse or physical therapist. The treating doctor will supply information, answer questions and dispel any myths to help provide the most positive yet realistic environment for motivating, energising and inspiring the patient to move forward on the road to a productive, useful life.

Family involvement becomes most important when the patient leaves hospital to be cared for at home. The patient's recovery will benefit greatly if the family provides encouragement, shows confidence in the patient's improvement, and permits them to do as much as they can and be as independent and vigorous as possible. The patient also needs to be reassured that they're wanted and needed and that they're still important to the family and part of the social picture.

It's important that the patient doesn't get too discouraged by their failures. They need to understand that many other people have recovered from a stroke and returned to normal activities or continued to do useful work. It's often helpful to give the recovering person manageable tasks, such as encouraging them to assume some household duties. It may also be useful to suggest that the patient take up new outside interests within their present capacities, particularly if they unable to return to work.

The stresses imposed on a family when someone has a stroke can be considerable, and many people find it difficult dealing with the emotional impact as well as the new responsibilities. This can sometimes lead to depression or anxiety. Family counselling and education in the form of individual sessions or through family support groups can be a big help in overcoming these problems.

What support is available for families and carers?

A stroke not only affects the patient but the whole family. It's always stressful for relatives to realise that their loved one has become disabled or might even die from the illness. Caring for a stroke patient at home can often lead to emotional, physical and financial strains. The more severe the disability after a stroke the more strain it puts on everyone concerned.

Before the patient is discharged from hospital, try to get a clear picture of their condition and probable recovery from the medical personnel. Also try to get answers to any questions you have about how to care for the patient at home.

You can also obtain information and support from local services, such as a district nurse, physiotherapist, occupational therapist, speech therapist, social worker, stroke services, caregiver support group or Needs Assessment Service Coordinator (see Recommended resources on pages 167–69 for contact details — this information is also available in some telephone directories and at local council offices).

It is important not to let the main caregiver become overwhelmed by their own problems and frustrations as this will affect both their health and the health of the person they are caring for. If you are the main caregiver, don't be afraid to ask for help or occasional time off. It's important that you try to maintain your outside interests and friendships. In most cases, it's possible to arrange alternative short-term care with a hospital or nursing home or with a family member or friend. In New Zealand, for example, there's the Carer Support Subsidy and the Respite Care Scheme to help caregivers. The Carer Support Subsidy provides short-term care for a stroke patient in a hospital, rest home or at home. The Respite Care Scheme provides temporary care in a rest home or private hospital for stroke patients with a high level of need.

Home carers can provide a range of supportive services, from intensive medical support to assistance with daily-living activities, housekeeping, meal preparation and transportation. Their help allows some patients with disabilities to remain in their own homes when they wouldn't otherwise be able to do so and also gives support to the caregivers. This care can be provided by nurses, social workers, occupational therapists, physiotherapists and other rehabilitation workers. The Stroke Foundation of New Zealand has field officers who liaise with health professionals, community agencies and volunteers to help stroke patients and their carers and families adjust to their changed circumstances with the ultimate purpose of improving their quality of life. These field officers are available to discuss any stroke-related problems, make hospital or home visits, advise on services available in the

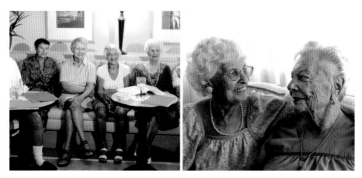

There are many different support groups for stroke patients and their carers.

community, liaise with Stroke Clubs and provide ongoing support to families. The Stroke Foundation of New Zealand also promotes stroke care, Stroke Clubs, rehabilitation, prevention, a network for young stroke patients, family support, spouse support groups, newsletters, and education and public awareness. In Stroke Clubs, people who've had a stroke meet regularly for mutual support and active participation in various social activities, such as bowls, exercise to music, table games, crafts and outings. The Younger Stroke Network provides support for younger people who've had a stroke and their caregivers. Caregiver Support Groups allow spouses and caregivers to meet, share their experiences and gain support from one another. These support groups may or may not be facilitated by an expert, and many are now available on-line via the Internet. The Stroke Centre of the Stroke Foundation provides information, brochures, reading material, books and videos. It also provides administration support and is the central point for the stroke community.

Is financial help available?

A stroke often affects the income of the patient and their family, especially if the patient has had to give up work. There may also be additional financial expenses related to organising care for the patient at home (e.g. paid nursing or social care, reduced working time for the family carer, purchasing new equipment for assisting the patient at home, etc.). The financial support available for stroke patients varies from country to country. In New Zealand, government-funded benefits and subsidies include accommodation support, carer support, provision of a community services card, a disability allowance, invalids' benefits, a living alone allowance, mobility vouchers (half-price taxi fares), national superannuation, residential care subsidy, respite care, sickness benefit, travel costs and other special grants.

> **AN EXAMPLE OF THE SERVICES PROVIDED BY THE STROKE FOUNDATION OF NEW ZEALAND**
>
> In August 2002, a woman in her sixties had a severe stroke, which affected the left side of her body. A field officer from the Stroke Foundation of New Zealand was informed about the woman's admission to hospital. She sent information about the available community services to the family caregiver. She also made phone contact, and arranged for a medical alarm to use in the house (these are free in New Zealand for people with community services cards) and for a mobility car sticker to give access to restricted parking. In addition, the patient was signed up for total mobility vouchers, which subsidise the cost of taxi fares, and a disability allowance, which helps towards doctors' fees, prescription fees, power bills, lawn mowing, gardening and any other costs incurred because of the stroke. When the patient was discharged, the field officer paid a home visit to discuss the patient's care and any other issues that had come up. She helped organise appointments at the outpatient clinic and checked the patient's referrals to community rehabilitation services. The family had had some problems with a medical alarm agent, so the field officer called the service and sorted it out. She also arranged for a Needs Assessment Service Coordinator to assess the family's need for home help. The patient joined her local Stroke Club and made good progress, improving physically and mentally. She still continues to improve and enjoy life.

Can someone drive a car after a stroke or TIA?

Each country has its own regulations concerning driving after a stroke or TIA. In New Zealand and Australia, a person should not drive until their clinical recovery is complete and there is no significant residual disability likely to compromise anyone's safety. However, this period shouldn't be less than

1 month after the event, and for people with residual deficits it should be no less than 3 months.

In general, the decision about driving is made by the patient's doctor, usually in consultation with an occupational therapist. The decision is based on an evaluation of the patient's vision, physical functioning (including coordination) and cognitive abilities. Things that will restrict someone from driving include: having had a seizure in the last 6 months; significant visual problems; ataxia; diplopia; recurrent TIAs; and significant cardiovascular disorders. People who've had recurrent TIAs shouldn't drive until the condition has been satisfactorily controlled with no further episodes for at least 3 months. Depending on their severity, the following conditions can also restrict a stroke patient from driving: marked memory problems, poor concentration, severe aphasia and neglect.

Is it possible to have sex after a stroke or TIA?

There's no medical reason for changing your sexual activity after either a stroke or a TIA. Although these conditions don't usually affect a person's ability to have sex, their sexual desire (libido) may wane because of the severity of the illness. Consult with a doctor before using any medications that increase erectile function, as stimulants such as these may increase the risk of a further stroke.

Some people with a physical disability find it difficult to have intercourse in the positions they used previously, and may need to find alternative positions, such as lying on the affected side. Some drug treatments can reduce the patient's libido and erectile function, however a doctor may be able to change the drugs or drug-treatment regimen to reduce these side effects.

Can I travel by aeroplane after a stroke or TIA?

Patients who've had a TIA should avoid air travel for 1 or 2 weeks after the event. For patients who've had a stroke this time is usually extended to 3–4 weeks, but may be even longer, depending on the person's medical condition and accompanying disorders. It's good idea to see a doctor before the flight to ensure that you're in a stable condition and to get advice on flying. During the flight, drink plenty of non-alcoholic drinks and periodically exercise your legs. If the flight is likely to take longer than four hours, it's best to plan a stopover if at all possible. Before any international air travel, notify your travel insurance company about the flight and your medical condition.

Can I get culturally specific care?

In the multi-cultural societies we now live in, there are many different perceptions of well-being and illness. Most health-care professionals are aware of the need to provide care suitable for people from different backgrounds to their own, and it should be possible to get care tailored to some extent to your own cultural perspective. In some cultures the extended family and community may want to be more or less involved in looking after a stroke patient and in their rehabilitation. It's important that you feel comfortable with letting the health professionals involved know what would suit you and your family best. If you have particular religious beliefs or traditional healing methods, don't be afraid to mention them when speaking to the patient's doctor. The aim is to work together with the health professionals to provide the best possible individual care and the most comfortable, familiar and supportive environment for the patient.

KEY INFORMATION

■ A stroke patient's recovery continues after they're discharged from hospital. Before going home, patients and their family members should be aware of the likely challenges ahead and have a clear understanding of the available community services.

■ The level of home care and rehabilitation needs to be tailored to the patient's condition and needs. Thorough everyday care and gradual rehabilitation can prevent serious complications and improve a patient's recovery after a stroke.

■ Patients should be encouraged to resume their previous activities as much as possible. Particular attention should be paid to the safety of the patient while they're performing these activities.

■ Family members and caregivers play a central role in the home care, rehabilitation and recovery of the patient. Culturally specific help and advice is often available.

■ There are special regulations about driving a car after a stroke or TIA that must be followed by all patients.

Concluding remarks

It's my hope that over the course of the book readers will have improved their understanding of stroke prevention, management and recovery. In particular, there are three important messages I want to convey.

Firstly, stroke is a highly preventable disorder that may be avoided by an overwhelming majority of people, but only if they recognise and adequately control their risk factors. Knowing your personal risk of having a stroke and dealing with your risk factors efficiently at the earliest possible stage are of paramount importance in preventing a stroke.

Secondly, stroke is an emergency, and modern management strategies are reasonably effective if adequate treatment is received in time. Early recognition of the warning signs of a stroke and emergency hospitalisation of the patient may not only be lifesaving but can substantially improve the chances of a good recovery.

Thirdly, a stroke, even a very severe stroke, isn't the end of the world for patients and their families as there's always potential for improvement. Although a debilitating stroke is frightening, patients and their families don't have to deal with it alone. There is variety of services to help and support them at personal, family and community levels. The capacity of the brain to recover from injuries, including a stroke, is enormous and not fully understood. Therefore stroke patients and their families should never give up their fight for recovery and better independence. Adequate care for a stroke patient and persistence in carrying out rehabilitation procedures are the keys to improvement.

Appendices

1 Common symptoms of a stroke by site of damage

The *right* or *left* hemisphere in the anterior (front) of the brain. Note: damage to either hemisphere affects the opposite side of body	The *right* hemisphere (in right-handed people) in the anterior of the brain	The *left* hemisphere (in right-handed people) in the anterior of the brain	Brain-stem and cerebellar strokes in the posterior of the brain
Partial or complete loss of strength in one side of the face or body	Loss of awareness of their right side (inc. denying existence of problem) and/or confusion between the left and right sides of body	Difficulty speaking and/or understanding what others are saying	Loss of movement on one side of the body and loss of sensation on the other side
Loss of feeling in one side of body	Slurred monotonous speech	Inability to read and/or write	Double vision
Loss of vision on the side opposite to the damage	Difficulty recognising familiar faces	Disconnected thoughts	Swallowing and/or speech difficulties
	Difficulty seeing how things relate to each other in space	Verbal memory loss (words)	Problems with balance and coordination
	Difficulty with abstract thinking (e.g. solving problems)	Poor motivation	Breathing problems (e.g. irregular breathing)
		Difficulty with even simple calculations	

2 Outline of a low-fat and low-cholesterol diet

Food	Any time	Sometimes	Avoid
Fruits and vegetables	Most fresh, juiced, frozen, canned or dried fruits and vegetables	Avocado, olives	Coconut; vegetables in cheese, cream or butter; fried or roasted vegetables
Grains (breads, cereals, pasta and baked goods)	Bread, bread-sticks, plain rolls, cereals, rice, bulgur wheat, pasta, fat-free and low-fat crackers and biscuits	Biscuits, muffins, waffles, French toast, unsalted popcorn, low-fat or reduced-fat snack foods	Doughnuts, croissants, sweet rolls, commercial egg noodles, stuffing, regular chips, crackers, pies, salted snack foods, cakes and biscuits
Dairy products	Trim milk, buttermilk, non-fat dry milk, fat-free yogurt and cheese, fat-free or low-fat cottage cheese	2% fat milk, 4% fat cottage cheese, reduced-fat and part-skim milk cheeses, low-fat yogurt, frozen yogurt	Whole milk, whole-milk yogurt and cheese, ice cream
Meat, eggs, and meat substitutes	Any fin fish or shellfish (except shrimp), poultry, ground turkey (without skin), select beef (round sirloin, tenderloin, flank, ground round), lamb (leg), pork (centre-cut ham, loin chops, tenderloin), low-fat luncheon meats, dried beans and peas, lentils, egg whites, tofu, soy meat substitutes, fat-free meat substitutes	Shrimp, oil-packed fish, fish sticks, poultry (with skin), ground beef (extra lean and lean), eggs (up to 4 per week)	Fried fish or poultry, pork or lamb (rib, brisket, shoulder, porterhouse, T-bone), organ (offal) meats, regular ground beef, sausage, bacon, most regular luncheon meats, peanut butter, nuts
Fats	Oils made from corn, sunflower, soybean, sesame, canola, olive or peanuts; margarine, reduced-fat margarine, reduced-fat salad dressing, fat-free sour cream	Regular salad dressing, mayonnaise, reduced-fat sour cream or cream cheese	Coconut oil, palm and palm kernel oils, shortening, lard, butter, cream, sour cream, cream cheese, gravy, most non-dairy creamers

3 Examples of healthy brain recipes

Adopted with permission from *Quick Food for the Heart* by G. Gourley, published by The National Heart Foundation of New Zealand, Penguin Books Ltd, Harmondsworth, Middlesex, England, 1999; and *Deliciously Healthy Cookbook* by The National Heart Foundation of Australia, R & R Publications Marketing Pty Ltd, Victoria, Australia, 2001, courtesy of the National Heart Foundation of New Zealand.

BREAKFAST

Bircher Muesli
(preparation time: 10 minutes + 1 hour standing; cooking time: nil)

1 apple, peeled, cored and grated
1 pear, peeled, cored and grated
2 cups rolled oats
½ tsp ground cinnamon
250 ml pear juice
150 g reduced-fat vanilla yogurt
50 g toasted flaked almonds
250 ml reduced-fat milk
2 mangoes, peeled and chopped
1 banana, sliced
2 passionfruit

Put the apple, pear, rolled oats, cinnamon and pear juice in a bowl and mix to combine. Allow to stand covered in the refrigerator for 1 hour.

Fold through the yogurt and almonds. Spoon the muesli into individual bowls and serve topped with the milk, mango and banana then drizzle with passionfruit pulp.

Serves 4

From *Deliciously Healthy Cookbook*

Skinny Eggs and Ham on Bagels
(preparation time: 20 minutes; cooking time: 5 minutes)

100 g cherry tomatoes
12 fresh flat parsley leaves
Canona cooking spray
4 eggs
4 egg whites
125 ml reduced-fat evaporated milk

ground white pepper to taste
2 wholemeal bagels, halved
100 g shaved reduced-fat ham

Cut the cherry tomatoes in half and place on a non-stick baking tray. Grill until soft and the skin begins to shrink. Remove and keep warm.

Put the parsley leaves on another baking tray, lightly spray with the oil and grill until crisp.

Put the egg, egg whites and evaporated milk in a bowl, whisk to combine and season with a little white pepper.

Pour the egg mixture into a non-stick frying pan and cook over a low heat until the egg starts to set. Stir gently until just cooked. Don't overcook or the texture will not be smooth.

Toast the four bagel halves, and top the bases with a little of the shaved ham, scrambled eggs, cherry tomatoes and crisp parsley leaves.

Serves 4

From *Deliciously Healthy Cookbook*

LUNCH

Cauliflower and Bean Salad

Note: Craisins are dried cranberries, which give this salad
a lovely colour and flavour.

1 tbsp oil
1 tsp finely grated lemon rind
¼ cup lemon juice
1 tbsp sugar
1 tbsp sherry (or water)
¼ cup craisins or currants
3 cups cauliflower florets
1–2 cups whole French beans
1 small red onion, finely sliced

Combine the oil, lemon rind and juice, sugar, sherry and craisins. Mix until sugar is completely dissolved. Blanch the cauliflower and beans in boiling water for 2–3 minutes. Cool under cold running water. Drain. Place in a bowl with the sliced onion and add the dressing. Mix gently until the vegetables are well coated in the dressing. Serve warm or cold.

Serves 4

From *Quick Food for the Heart*

Tomato and Basil Salad

4–6 tomatoes, sliced
1–2 red onions, finely sliced into rings
1 cup fresh basil leaves
¼ cup spiced vinegar
2 tbsp oil
1 tsp sugar
freshly ground black pepper

Layer the tomatoes, onions and basil on a serving platter. Place the vinegar, oil and sugar in a screw-top jar and shake until the sugar dissolves. Pour over the salad. Season generously with the pepper.

Serves 4

From *Quick Food for the Heart*

Panini with Brie, Chicken and Stonefruit

1 panini bread
40 g sliced brie or camembert
¼ cup chopped cooked or smoked chicken, skin removed
½ cup sliced raw or canned apricot, peach, nectarine or plum

Toast the panini bread in a toaster, under the grill, on the barbecue or even in a 'dry' frying pan until lightly golden and crusty.

Split, pile in the brie, chicken and fruit.

From *Quick Food for the Heart*

DINNER

Vegetable and Chickpea Curry with Poppy Seed Rice
(preparation time: 30 minutes; cooking time: 25 minutes)

2 tbsp soybean oil
1 brown onion, thinly sliced
1 tbsp grated fresh ginger
3 cloves garlic, crushed
3 long green chillies, finely chopped
½ tsp ground turmeric
2 tsp ground coriander
2 tsp garam masala
2 potatoes, cut into large cubes
2 carrots, cut into thick slices
2 zucchini, cut into thick slices
425 g can chopped tomatoes
250 ml reduced-salt vegetable stock

400 g can chickpeas, rinsed and drained
200 g baby spinach leaves, washed
1 cup fresh or frozen peas
poppy seed rice (1½ cups basmati rice, 2 tbsp poppy seeds)
2 microwave poppadoms to serve

Heat the oil in a large pot, add the onion and ginger and cook over a medium heat for 5 minutes or until soft. Add the garlic, chillies and spices and cook for 2 minutes or until fragrant.

Add the potatoes and carrots and cook until the vegetables are coated in the spices. Stir in the zucchini, tomatoes and stock and simmer. Reduce the heat and cook for 15 minutes or until the vegetables are tender and the curry has thickened slightly. Add the chickpeas and stir.

Add the spinach leaves and peas; cook just until the spinach wilts and the peas are soft.

To make the poppy seed rice, put the rice and poppy seeds in a pot, add 450 ml of water and bring to the boil. Cook over a high heat until tunnels appear in the rice. Reduce the heat to very low, cover and allow to steam for 10 minutes or until the rice is tender and all the liquid is absorbed.

Serve the curry on top of the rice and accompany with microwave poppadoms.

Serves 4

From *Deliciously Healthy Cookbook*

Steamed Fish Rolls with Tomato Vinaigrette
(preparation time: 20 minutes; cooking time: 10 minutes)

4 (about 700 g) boneless, skinless white fish fillets
2 tbsp grape seed oil
2 cloves garlic, crushed
6 spring onions, chopped
1 cup fresh wholemeal breadcrumbs
½ cup fresh basil leaves, chopped
1 cup fresh flat leaf parsley, chopped
1 tsp lemon zest
2 tbsp lemon juice
250 ml tomato juice
2 tbsp white wine vinegar
1 tbsp brown sugar

Cut the fish fillets in half lengthwise, following the natural centre line

Heat 1 tbsp of the oil in a large non-stick frying pan, add the garlic and spring onions and cook over a medium heat for 3 minutes or until the spring onions are soft. Put in a food processor with the breadcrumbs, half the basil, half the parsley and the lemon zest and juice. Process to combine.

Divide the stuffing into eight equal portions and roll into oblong shapes; put a piece on the end of each piece of fish and roll up to enclose the filling. Secure the rolls with a toothpick or piece of string. Cover and refrigerate for 30 minutes.

Finely chop the remaining basil and parsley and put into a saucepan with the tomato juice, vinegar and brown sugar. Cook over a low heat until warm.

Put the fresh rolls in a large bamboo steamer lined with baking paper. Cover and put over a wok of simmering water, making sure the base of the steamer doesn't touch the water. Steam for 10 minutes or until the fish is tender and the stuffing heated through.

Serve the fish rolls drizzled with tomato vinaigrette and a crisp green salad.

Serves 4

From *Deliciously Healthy Cookbook*

4 Recommended weights for adults

RECOMMENDED WEIGHTS
BASED ON BODY MASS INDEX (BMI)

Adopted from the New Zealand Food for Health and Nutrition Task Force Report 1991.

Height		Weight — Adults 20–60 years		Weight — Adult 60+ years	
(cm)	(feet and inches)*	(kg)	(lb)†	(kg)	(lb)†
160	5.3	51–64	113–141	51–72	113–158
162	5.4	53–66	116–144	53–74	116–162
164	5.5	54–67	118–147	54–75	118–165
166	5.5	55–69	121–152	55–77	121–170
168	5.6	56–71	124–155	56–79	124–174
170	5.7	58–72	127–159	58–81	127–177
172	5.7	60–74	130–163	59–83	130–182
174	5.8	61–76	133–167	61–85	133–187
176	5.9	62–77	136–170	62–87	136–191
178	5.10	63–79	139–174	63–89	139–195
180	5.11	65–81	142–178	65–91	142–200
182	5.11	66–83	146–182	66–93	146–204
184	6.0	68–85	149–186	68–95	149–209

*1 m = 39.37 inches; 1 inch = 2.54 cm   † 1 kg = 2.20 lb; 1 lb = 0.45 kg

BODY MASS INDEX (BMI) AND RISK OF ASSOCIATED DISORDERS

BMI (kg/m²), (lb/inch²)* weight in kg

Height in m

(The chart plots BMI values for weight in kg across the top (50–150) against height in m down the side (1.48–1.94), with cells colour-coded by classification.)

Colour key: Underweight · Normal range · Overweight · Obese 1 · Obese 2 · Obese 3

CLASSIFICATION OF WEIGHT BY BMI IN ADULT EUROPEANS		
CLASSIFICATION	BMI (kg/m²)	RISK OF CO-MORBIDITIES
Underweight	< 18.5	Low (but increased risk of other medical problems)
Normal range	18.5 – 24.9	Average
Overweight (pre-obese)	25 – 29.9	Increased
Obese 1	30 – 34.9	Moderate
Obese 2	35 – 39.9	Severe
Obese 3	> 40	Very severe

*Adopted from World Health Organisation 'Prevention and management of the global epidemic of obesity', Geneva 3–5 June 1997

5 Sample layout of a stroke patient's diary*

Keep a simplified diary to register a patient's details including medication and appointment times with health-care professionals.

Name _____

Address _____

Phone _____

Contact person(s) _____

Family members _____

Pets _____

Favourite pastimes _____

This stroke happened on _____

Diagnosis _____

Hospital _____ Ward _____

Admitted _____

Discharged (date) _____ to _____

Recommended medication to take	Dosage	Time taken	Purpose of drug
1 _____	_____	_____	_____
2 _____	_____	_____	_____
3 _____	_____	_____	_____
4 _____	_____	_____	_____
5 _____	_____	_____	_____
6 _____	_____	_____	_____
7 _____	_____	_____	_____
8 _____	_____	_____	_____
9 _____	_____	_____	_____
10 _____	_____	_____	_____

Discharge plan

District nurse to call ＿＿ days a week

Referred to ＿＿＿＿＿＿＿＿＿＿＿＿＿

Field Officer will call ＿＿＿＿＿＿＿＿＿＿＿＿＿

Meals on Wheels from ＿＿＿＿＿＿＿＿＿＿＿＿

Social worker ＿＿＿＿＿＿＿＿＿＿＿＿＿＿＿

Transport ＿＿＿＿＿＿＿＿＿＿＿＿＿

See family doctor on ＿＿＿＿＿＿＿＿＿＿＿＿＿＿＿＿

Other appointments:	*Day*	*Time*
Physiotherapy		
＿＿＿＿＿＿＿＿	＿＿＿	＿＿＿
＿＿＿＿＿＿＿＿	＿＿＿	＿＿＿
＿＿＿＿＿＿＿＿	＿＿＿	＿＿＿
＿＿＿＿＿＿＿＿	＿＿＿	＿＿＿
Occupational therapy		
＿＿＿＿＿＿＿＿	＿＿＿	＿＿＿
＿＿＿＿＿＿＿＿	＿＿＿	＿＿＿
＿＿＿＿＿＿＿＿	＿＿＿	＿＿＿
Speech-language therapy		
＿＿＿＿＿＿＿＿	＿＿＿	＿＿＿
＿＿＿＿＿＿＿＿	＿＿＿	＿＿＿
＿＿＿＿＿＿＿＿	＿＿＿	＿＿＿
＿＿＿＿＿＿＿＿	＿＿＿	＿＿＿

Occupational therapist's recommendations (following home visit):

＿＿＿＿＿＿＿＿＿＿＿＿＿＿＿＿＿＿＿＿＿＿＿＿＿

＿＿＿＿＿＿＿＿＿＿＿＿＿＿＿＿＿＿＿＿＿＿＿＿＿

＿＿＿＿＿＿＿＿＿＿＿＿＿＿＿＿＿＿＿＿＿＿＿＿＿

＿＿＿＿＿＿＿＿＿＿＿＿＿＿＿＿＿＿＿＿＿＿＿＿＿

*Modified with kind permission from the Stroke Foundation of New Zealand

6   Goals and results*

It's a good idea to keep a record of a stroke patient's progress either by writing or with photographs or videotape. If this isn't possible, progress can be measured using symbols: + for noticeable improvement, 0 for no change, and – for worsening.

Date	Target	To be achieved by	Results (total and by days)									
			1	2	3	4	5	6	7	8	9	etc
Speech therapist	Main goal:											
	Sub-goals:											
Physio-therapist	Main goal:											
	Sub-goals:											
Occupational therapist	Main goal:											
	Sub-goals:											
Personal	Main goal:											
	Sub-goals:											

*Modified with kind permission from the Stroke Foundation of New Zealand

RECOMMENDED RESOURCES

COMMUNITY CONTACTS IN NEW ZEALAND
The Stroke Foundation of New Zealand
Telephone: 0800 STROKE (787653)
Website: www.stroke.org.nz
Email: strokenz@stroke.org.nz
Evidence-based stroke guidelines: www.nzgg.org.nz

COMMUNITY CONTACTS IN AUSTRALIA
National Stroke Foundation
Suite 304, Level 3, 167–169 Queen Street, Melbourne, VIC 3000
Telephone: 03 9670 1000
Fax: 03 9670 9300
Freecall: 1800 STROKE (787653)
Website: www.strokefoundation.com.au
Email: admin@strokefoundation.com.au

COMMUNITY CONTACTS IN THE UK
Stroke Association: Stroke House
240 City Road, London EC1V 2PR
Telephone: 020 7566 0300
Fax: 020 7490 2686
Helpline: 0845 30 33 100
Website: www.stroke.org.uk
Email: info@stroke.org.uk

Chest, Heart and Stroke Scotland
65 North Castle Street, Edinburgh EH2 3LT
Telephone: 0131 225 6963
Fax: 0131 220 6313
Website: www.chss.org.uk
Email: admin@chss.org.uk

Northern Ireland Chest, Heart and Stroke Association
22 Great Victoria Street, Belfast BT2 7LX
Telephone: 028 9032 0184
Fax: 028 9033 3487
Helpline: 028 9026 6710
Website: www.nichsa.com
Email: mail@nichsa.com

To find out more information from the Stroke Association or to find the nearest information point for your area in the UK, see the website: www.stroke.org.uk/county.htm

COMMUNITY CONTACTS IN THE USA
American Stroke Association
7272 Greenville Avenue, Dallas, Texas 75231
Telephone: 888 4 STROKE (787653), 888 478 7653
Website: www.strokeassociation.org
Email: strokeinfo@heart.org

National Family Caregivers Association
10400 Connecticut Avenue, #500, Kensington,
Maryland 20895-3944
Telephone: 800 896 3650
Fax: 301 942 2302
Website: www.nfcacares.org
Email: info@nfcacares.org

National Stroke Association
9707 East Easter Lane, Englewood, Colorado 80112-3747
Telephone: 303 649 9299, 800 STROKES (7876537)
Fax: 303 649 1328
Website: www.stroke.org
Email: info@stroke.org

Stroke Clubs International
805 12th Street, Galveston, Texas 77550
Telephone: 409 762 1022
Email: strokeclub@earthlink.net

To find out more information from the American Stroke
Association or to find the nearest information point for your
area in the USA, see the website: local.strokeassociation.org

COMMUNITY CONTACTS IN CANADA
Heart and Stroke Foundation of Canada
222 Queen Street, Suite 1402, Ottawa, Ontario K1P 5V9
Telephone: 613 569 4361
Fax: 613 569 3278
Website: ww2.heartandstroke.ca

To find out more information from the Heart and Stroke
Foundation of Canada or to find the nearest information
point for your area in Canada, see the website:
ww2.heartandstroke.ca/Page.asp?PageID=97#Info

COMMUNITY CONTACTS IN SOUTH AFRICA
The National Heart Foundation
PO Box 15139, Vlaeberg 8018
Telephone: 021 447 4222
Fax: 021 447 0322
Website: www.heartfoundation.co.za
Email: heart@heartfoundation.co.za

To find out more information from the National Heart
Foundation or to find the nearest information point for your
area in South Africa, see the website:
www.heartfoundation.co.za/contact.php

SUGGESTED FURTHER READING

J. Baskett. *Life after Stroke: A guide for people with a stroke and their families.* Stroke Foundation of New Zealand Inc., Wellington, 1998.

G. Donnan and C. Burton. *After a Stroke: A Support Book for Patients, Caregivers, Families and Friends.* North Atlantic Books, Berkeley, California, 1992.

D.M. Hinds. *After Stroke. The Complete, Step-by-Step Blueprint for Getting Better.* Thorsons, London, 2000.

C. Hutton and L.R. Caplan. *Striking Back at Stroke: A Doctor-Patient Journal.* The DANA Press, Washington, D.C., 2003.

D.O. Wiebers. *Stroke-Free for Life. The Complete Guide to Stroke Prevention and Treatment.* HarperCollins*Publishers*, Inc., New York, New York, 2002.

D.O. Wiebers, V.L. Feigin, R.D. Brown Jr. *Cerebrovascular Disease in Clinical Practice.* Little, Brown and Company, Boston, 1997.

D.O. Wiebers, V.L. Feigin, R.D. Brown Jr. *Handbook of Stroke.* Lippincott-Raven Publishers, Philadelphia, 1997.

GLOSSARY OF STROKE TERMS

acute stroke — a stage starting at the onset of the stroke symptoms and lasting for a few hours

agnosia — impairment of the ability to recognise, or comprehend the meaning of, some sensory stimuli (e.g. colour, sight, touch, position)

agraphia — inability to write

alexia — inability to read

aneurysm — a weak spot in the artery wall that balloons out

aneurysm clipping — a surgical procedure for the treatment of brain aneurysms, involving clamping an aneurysm from a blood vessel

angiography — an X-ray of blood vessels after the injection of a contrast substance that shows up on an X-ray image

anosognosia — the lack of awareness or denial of a disease (e.g. a patient denies there is anything wrong with one side of their body)

anticoagulants — drugs used to prevent the formation or growth of blood clots by inhibiting the coagulation of the blood protein thrombin; some common anticoagulants include heparin and warfarin

antiplatelet agents — drugs used to prevent the formation or growth of blood clots by inhibiting the accumulation of platelets in the blood; some common antiplatelet agents include aspirin, plavix and aggrenox

antithrombotics — a generic term related to either anticoagulants or antiplatelet agents

aphasia — inability to understand or create speech

apoplexy — an old Latin term for a stroke defined as 'a stroke of God's hands'

apoptosis — a form of programmed, genetically triggered cell death involving shrinking of the cell and eventual disposal of the internal elements of the cell by the body's immune system

apraxia — inability to perform skilled or purposeful voluntary movements even though the person is physically able to do so

arrhythmia — an irregular heartbeat

arteriography — an X-ray of the arteries after the injection of a contrast substance that shows up on an X-ray image

arteriovenous malformation (AVM) — a congenital disorder (present at birth) characterised by a complex tangled web of arteries and veins

artery — a blood vessel that carries blood away from the heart

aspiration — the act of inhaling solid or liquid materials into the lungs

aspiration pneumonia — a chest infection (pneumonia) caused by inhaling foreign material, usually food particles or vomit, into the lungs

asteriognosis — inability to identify an object by touch

ataxia — lack of coordination, unsteadiness

atheroma — a mixture of fatty substances, including cholesterol and other lipids, deposited on the inside of an artery wall (synonym: plaque)

atherosclerosis — a disease of the arteries characterised by deposits of fats that make the arteries hard, thick (narrow) and brittle; the terms atherosclerosis and arteriosclerosis are often used interchangeably

atrial fibrillation — irregular beating of the left atrium, or left-upper chamber, of the heart

bilateral — both sides of the body

blood-brain barrier — an elaborate meshwork that surrounds the blood vessels and capillaries in the brain and regulates which elements in the blood can pass through to the neurons (brain cells)

brain stem — the stem-like, lower part of the brain that connects the brain's right and left hemispheres with the spinal cord

brain stem stroke — a stroke that strikes the brain stem

capillaries — the tiniest blood vessels in the body, from which oxygen and nutrients pass into the surrounding body tissues, and carbon dioxide and waste products are removed from the tissues to the veins

cardiac — relating to the heart

cardiovascular — relating to the heart and blood vessels

caregivers — individuals (often family members or friends) who provide assistance to see that the physical, psychological and social needs of another person are met; they are often unpaid

carotid artery — one of two arteries, located on either side of the neck, that carry blood to the brain

carotid endarterectomy — an operation to remove atheromas from a narrowed carotid artery (usually the internal carotid artery)

carotid stenosis — narrowing of the carotid artery

catheter — a medical device (a tube and receptacle bag) used to control urinary incontinence

central pain — pain caused by damage to an area in the mid-brain called the thalamus

cerebellar stroke — a stroke that strikes the cerebellum

cerebellum — the part of the brain at the back that is responsible for coordinating voluntary muscle movements

cerebral — relating to the brain

cerebral blood flow (CBF) — the flow of blood through the arteries that lead to the brain

cerebral cortex — the outer layer of the brain

cerebral haemorrhage — bleeding into the brain tissue (intracerebral haemorrhage) or into the surrounding areas (subarachnoid haemorrhage)

cerebral hemisphere — one of the two halves of the brain

cerebral infarct — an area where brain cells have died (synonym: ischaemic stroke)

cerebral oedema — swelling of the brain

cerebral thrombosis — the closing off of an artery in the brain by a blood clot

cerebrovascular accident (CVA) — an old term used for a stroke, which is falling into disuse because a stroke is no longer viewed as an accident

cerebrovascular disease (CVD) — encompasses all abnormalities in the brain resulting from problems with the blood vessels (e.g. narrowing or a blockage)

cholesterol — a waxy substance, produced naturally by the liver and also found in foods, that circulates in the blood

cognition — higher intellectual (mental) functioning associated with thinking, learning, perception and memory

cognitive impairment — a deficiency in a person's thinking, judgment, short- or long-term memory or knowledge of where they are, the time or the people around them

coma — a state of deep unconsciousness where the person is not responsive or able to be aroused

compensation — the ability of a person with impairments from a stroke to perform a task (or tasks) either using the impaired limb with an adapted approach or using the unaffected limb to perform the task

computerised tomography (CT) **scan** — a series of cross-sectional X-rays of the brain and head; previously called computerised axial tomography (CAT)

confabulation — filling gaps in the memory with imagined events

continence — the ability to control bladder and bowel functions

contracture — static muscle shortening; the muscle cannot be lengthened and there is loss of motion in the adjacent joint

contralateral — the opposite side of the body

coordination — the harmonious working together of several muscles or muscle groups in the execution of complex movements

dementia — loss of intellectual ability (e.g. vocabulary, abstract thinking, judgment, memory, physical coordination) that interferes with daily activities

depression — a reversible psychiatric disorder characterised by an inability to concentrate, difficulty sleeping, feelings of hopelessness, fatigue, the 'blues' and guilt

diplopia — double vision

duplex carotid scan — an ultrasound scan of the carotid arteries in the neck

dysarthria — a motor disorder of the tongue, mouth, jaw or voice-box resulting in difficulty in producing speech

dyslexia — difficulty with reading

dyslipidaemia — abnormality in the blood lipids (fats)

dysphagia — inability to swallow or difficulty swallowing

dysphasia — difficulty understanding or creating speech

dysphonia — impairment of the voice

dyspraxia — difficulty performing skilled or purposeful voluntary movements even though the person is physically able to do so

echocardiogram — an ultrasound scan of the heart

electrocardiogram (ECG) — a graph that displays the electrical activity and rhythm of the heart

electroencephalogram (EEG) — a graph that displays the electrical activity in the brain by placing electrodes on the scalp

embolic stroke — a stroke caused by an embolus

embolism — blockage of a blood vessel by an embolus

embolus — a blood clot that travels in the bloodstream

emotional lability — a condition in which the mood of the person swings rapidly from one state to another (such as laughing, crying or anger) for no obvious external reason

enteral feeding — feeding via a tube connecting with the stomach

epidemiology — the study of the factors that influence the frequency and distribution of a disease in a population

epilepsy — a condition resulting in seizures, or fits, involving the whole body or parts of it

extracranial-intracranial (EC-IC) bypass — a type of surgery that restores blood flow to a blood-deprived area of brain tissue by re-routing a healthy artery in the scalp to the area of brain tissue affected by a blocked or narrowed artery

gait — manner of walking

geriatrician — a doctor who specialises in the care of older people, primarily those who are frail and have complex medical or social problems

glia — the supportive cells of the nervous system, which play an important role in brain functioning (synonym: neuroglia)

haematoma — a collection of blood forming a definite swelling that compresses and damages the brain around it

haemorrhage — bleeding

haemorrhagic — relating to bleeding

haemorrhagic stroke — bleeding into the brain (intracerebral haemorrhage) or into surrounding areas (subarachnoid haemorrhage)

hemianaesthesia — loss of sensation on one side of the body

hemianopia — loss of half the field of vision in each eye

hemi-inattention — lack of awareness of what's happening on one side of the body (synonym: unilateral neglect)

hemiparesis — weakness on one side of the body

hemiplegia — complete paralysis on one side of the body

hemisphere — one half of the brain (synonym: cerebral hemisphere)

hemispheric stroke — a stroke that strikes one of the brain's hemispheres

heparin — a type of anticoagulant

high-density lipoprotein cholesterol (HDL-C) — a compound consisting of a lipid (a fat) and a protein, it carries cholesterol in the blood and deposits it in the liver; also known as the 'good' cholesterol

home care — a range of supportive services in the home from intensive medical support to assistance with daily-living activities and housekeeping

hypertension — abnormally high blood pressure

hypotension — abnormally low blood pressure

impairment — a physical or mental defect at the level of a body system or organ

impotence — inability to obtain or maintain penile erection

incidence — describes the frequency with which cases of a disease occur during a certain period of time in a population

incontinence — inability to control bladder (urinary incontinence) or bowel functions (bowel incontinence) or both

infarct or **infarction** — an area of dead or dying tissue

intracerebral haemorrhage — bleeding into the brain

intravenous — in a vein

involuntary — bodily actions that happen without being willed or intended

ischaemia — a loss or reduction of blood flow to body tissue

ischaemic cascade — a series of pathophysiological and biochemical events lasting from several hours to several days following an initial ischaemia

ischaemic penumbra — area of damaged, but still living, brain cells arranged in a patchwork pattern around areas of dead brain cells

ischaemic stroke — a stroke caused by a blockage or narrowing of one or more arteries leading to the brain

lacunar infarction — a small area of dead brain often caused by stenosis or occlusion of the small arteries in the brain

large artery disease — stenosis or occlusion of the carotid arteries, often caused by atherosclerosis

lipoprotein — small globules of cholesterol covered by a layer of protein

low-density lipoprotein cholesterol (LDL-C) — a compound consisting of a lipid (a fat) and a protein, it carries cholesterol in the blood and deposits the excess along the inside of arterial walls; also known as the 'bad' cholesterol

magnetic resonance angiography (MRA) — a technique that involves injecting a contrast substance into a blood vessel and using magnetic resonance to create an image of the arteries and veins in the brain

magnetic resonance imaging (MRI) scan — a type of brain imaging involving the use of a powerful magnetic field to generate and measure interactions between pulsed magnetic waves and hydrogen nuclei (such as those in water) within the tissues of the head

monoparesis — weakness in one limb only

monoplegia — paralysis in one limb only

mortality rate — the number of people who die during a certain period of time

motor — relating to movement in the body

nasogastric tube — a tube put down the nose into the stomach

neglect, one-sided — a term sometimes used for lack of awareness on one side of the body

neuron — a brain cell or nerve cell, the main functional unit of the brain and nervous system; a single neuron is a long elongated cell that receives and passes on impulses to other neurons

neuroprotective agents — medications that protect the brain from injury

nursing home — a generic term for a skilled nursing facility

oedema — swelling

orthosis — an external orthopaedic device, such as a brace or splint, that prevents or assists movement of the spine or the limbs

paraesthesia — an abnormal sensation, such as feeling of burning, pricking, tickling or tingling, without an obvious cause

paraparesis — weakness in both legs (can result from bilateral strokes or spinal cord problems)

paraphrasia — producing unintended phrases, words or syllables during speech

paraplegia — paralysis of both legs (can result from bilateral strokes or spinal cord problems)

paresis — muscle weakness

PEG tube — a percutaneous endoscopic gastrostomy feeding tube, which is inserted through the abdominal wall into the stomach

perception — the ability to receive, interpret and use information

plaque — a mixture of fatty substances, including cholesterol and other lipids, deposited on inside of an artery wall (synonym: atheroma)

plasticity of the brain — the ability of the brain to adapt to deficits and injury by intact cells taking over functions of damaged ones

platelets — blood cells with a role in blood coagulation

rehabilitation — restoration of a disabled person to their greatest possible independence

rest home — a group home, specialised apartment complex or other institution that provides live-in care services; sometimes referred to as a private hospital, residential care facility or a care home

silent stroke — a stroke the produces no obvious symptoms

small artery disease — a disease of the small arteries in the brain, often caused by hypertension

spasm — involuntary contraction of a muscle

spastic paralysis — paralysis with increased muscle tone and spasmodic contraction of the muscles

spasticity — abnormally increased tone in a muscle

stenosis — narrowing

stroke — an acute vascular injury of the brain

stroke unit — a hospital facility for the management of stroke patients by a multi-disciplinary team of specialists

subarachnoid haemorrhage — bleeding between the brain surface and one of the thin layers of tissue that cover the brain

tactile — relating to touch

thromboembolus — a clot that has travelled in an artery or vein

thrombolytics — drugs that dissolve blood clots

thrombosis — the formation of a blood clot

thrombotic stroke — a stroke caused by thrombosis

thrombus — a blood clot

tinnitus — 'ringing' in the ears

tone — the degree of tension in a muscle at rest

total serum cholesterol — a combined measurement of a person's high-density lipoprotein cholesterol (HDL-C) and low-density lipoprotein cholesterol (LDL-C)

transcranial magnetic stimulation (TMS) — a small magnetic current delivered to an area of the brain to promote plasticity and healing

transient ischaemic attack (TIA) — a short-lived stroke that lasts from a few minutes to 24 hours; often called a mini stroke or a minor stroke

vascular — relating to the blood vessels

vasospasm — spasm of a blood vessel; a dangerous side effect of a subarachnoid haemorrhage

vein — a blood vessel that carries blood back to the heart

vertebral arteries — two arteries on either side of the back of the neck within the bones of the spine that carry blood to the brain

vertebrobasilar arteries — the two arteries on the back of the neck that supply blood to the brain stem and cerebellum

videofluoroscopy — a video X-ray of a person's swallowing mechanism

visuospatial disorder — inability to recognise or perceive time, distance or areas of space

whanau — a Maori word meaning the extended family

INDEX

A

activity of daily living (daily
activity)
  improvement of 40, 52,
    54, 133, 139
  stroke effects on 82, 133
aerobic exercise 54, 139
African Americans, risk of
  stroke 26
age, ageing
  and recovery from a stroke
    88, 89, 94
  as a stroke risk factor 20,
    21, 25, 26, 28, 33, 39, 51
  stroke prevention and 59, 85
aids
  home 95, 113, 125, 138
  incontinence 95, 129, 130,
    176
  walking 137
alcohol
  as a stroke risk factor 30, 38
  consumption of 31
  binge drinking 30
  control of 54, 55
  excess of 19
  haemorrhagic strokes and 30
  ischaemic strokes and 30
  stroke prevention and 54
American stroke societies 168
aneurysms
  and haemorrhagic strokes
    14, 15
  and risk of a stroke 19
  intracranial 8, 15
  ruptured 16
  smoking and 29

stroke prevention and 28, 51
unruptured 27, 51
angina
  ischaemic heart disease 21,
    34
  stroke prevention and 74
angiography 51, 71–73
angiotensin converting
  enzyme (ACE) inhibitors 45
antiarrhythmic agents 47
antibiotics 130
anticoagulants (blood thinners)
  as a haemorrhagic stroke
    cause 87
  factors that affect 88
  for an ischaemic stroke 87
  for artery blockage or
    stenosis 87
  for atrial fibrillation 47
  for prevention of recurrent
    strokes 86
antidepressant medications
  57, 141
antihypertensive medications
  45, 46
antiplatelet agents
  for artery blockage or
    stenosis 87
  for prevention of recurrent
    strokes 87, 88
anxiety 146
appetite 34, 42, 124
arteries
  blockage of 7, 8, 12, 24
  disease of 23
  inflammation of 14, 35
  stenosis of 24, 48